THE COMPLETE
EYE HEALTH &
NUTRITION GUIDE

eyefoods®

Laurie Capogna, OD

Robert
ROSE

Eyefoods
Text copyright © 2019 Laurie Capogna
Cover and text design copyright © 2019 Robert Rose Inc.

For complete cataloguing information, see page 240.

Disclaimer

This book is a general guide only and should never be a substitute for the skill, knowledge and experience of a qualified medical professional dealing with the facts, circumstances and symptoms of a particular case.

The nutritional, medical and health information presented in this book is based on the research, training and professional experience of the author, and is true and complete to the best of her knowledge. However, this book is intended only as an informative guide for those wishing to know more about eye health, nutrition and medicine; it is not intended to replace or countermand the advice given by the reader's personal physician. Because each person and situation is unique, the author and the publisher urge the reader to check with a qualified health-care professional before using any procedure where there is a question as to its appropriateness. The author and the publisher are not responsible for any adverse effects or consequences resulting from the use of the information in this book. It is the responsibility of the reader to consult a physician or other qualified health-care professional regarding their personal care.

This book contains references to products that may not be available everywhere. The intent of the information provided is to be helpful; however, there is no guarantee of results associated with the information provided. Use of brand names is for educational purposes only and does not imply endorsement.

The recipes in this book have been carefully tested by our kitchen and our tasters. To the best of our knowledge, they are safe and nutritious for ordinary use and users. For those people with food or other allergies, or who have special food requirements or health issues, please read the suggested contents of each recipe carefully and determine whether or not they may create a problem for you. All recipes are used at the risk of the consumer. We cannot be responsible for any hazards, loss or damage that may occur as a result of any recipe use. For those with special needs, allergies, requirements or health problems, in the event of any doubt, please contact your medical adviser prior to the use of any recipe.

At the time of publication, all URLs referenced link to existing websites. Robert Rose Inc. is not responsible for maintaining, and does not endorse the content of, any website or content not created by Robert Rose Inc.

Design and production: Daniella Zanchetta/PageWave Graphics Inc.
Editor: Sue Sumeraj
Recipe editor: Jennifer MacKenzie
Proofreader: Kelly Jones
Indexer: Gillian Watts

Front cover images: carrot © iStockphoto.com/Floortje; variety of healthy food items © iStockphoto.com/dulezidar; yellow pepper © iStockphoto.com/baibaz; orange pepper © iStockphoto.com/kyoshino; kiwi © iStockphoto.com/Creativeye99; eggs © iStockphoto.com/Bozena_Fulawka
Back cover/spine images: bowl of kale © iStockphoto.com/Karaidel; orange pepper © iStockphoto.com/kyoshino
Interior images: p. 29 swan © iStockphoto.com/Basmeelker; p. 39 sunflower © iStockphoto.com/Allusioni
Illustrations: p. 11, p. 15 eye anatomy and p. 12 visual process © Margaret Amy Salter

The publisher gratefully acknowledges the financial support of our publishing program by the Government of Canada through the Canada Book Fund.

Canadä

Published by Robert Rose Inc.
120 Eglinton Avenue East, Suite 800, Toronto, Ontario, Canada M4P 1E2
Tel: (416) 322-6552 Fax: (416) 322-6936
www.robertrose.ca

Printed and bound in Canada

1 2 3 4 5 6 7 8 9 MI 27 26 25 24 23 22 21 20 19

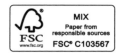

Contents

Introduction 4

PART 1: EYE HEALTH AND DISEASE

Chapter 1: Eye Anatomy and Vision 8
Eye Anatomy. 8
The Visual Process. 12
Refractive Errors 13
Eye Nutrition Basics. 14

**Chapter 2: Taking Care of Your Eyes,
Decade by Decade. 16**
In the First 10 Years 16
Tweens and Teens 19
In Your 20s and 30s 20
In Your 40s and 50s 21
In Your 60s and 70s 23
In Your 80s, 90s and Beyond 25

**Chapter 3: Common Eye Conditions
and Diseases. 28**
Age-Related Macular Degeneration . . . 29
Cataracts. 38
Dry Eye Syndrome. 41
Eyelid Disorders 50
Glaucoma. 52
Diabetes and Eye Health. 61

PART 2: THE EYEFOODS PLAN

Chapter 4: Eye Nutrients 68
Macronutrients and General Health . . . 68
Micronutrients and General Health 73
Top Nutrients for Eye Health. 74

Chapter 5: Eyefoods. 83
Leafy Green Vegetables 83
Cold-Water Fish. 87
Orange Vegetables 90
Orange Bell Peppers. 92
Green Vegetables 93
Eggs 94

Fruit and Fruit Juice 95
Lean Protein. 96
Nuts and Seeds 98
Whole Grains 99
Beans and Lentils. 102
Healthy Fats 104

**Chapter 6: Lifestyle and
General Health 105**
Ultraviolet and Blue Light Exposure. . .105
Smoking. 110
Body Mass Index and Waist
Circumference 110
Physical Activity 111

**Chapter 7: Following the
Eyefoods Plan. .112**
Weekly Targets. 112
Serving Sizes. 114
The Eyefoods Nutrition Plan 115
The Eyefoods Lifestyle Plan. 116
If You Follow a Paleo Diet. 117
If You Follow a Plant-Based Diet. 118

**Chapter 8: Integrating Eyefoods
into Your Diet .120**
Track It! 121
Sample Weekly Meal Plans 122
Pantry and Freezer Lists. 124

PART 3: RECIPES FOR HEALTHY EYES
Breakfasts. 126
Smoothies and Juices. 135
Salads and Dressings 151
Starters, Side Dishes and Sauces 175
Main Courses 189
Healthy Snacks and Desserts 221

Resources and References. 230
Index. 235

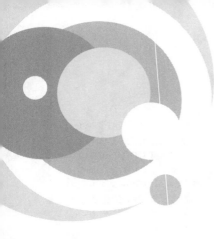

Introduction

This book is for everyone who wants to learn more about eye health and the prevention of eye disease. I have taken the experience I have gained in my 20 years of optometric practice, integrated it with the most up-to-date scientific research and developed a list of the best foods for helping us maintain healthy eyes and vision and prevent certain eye diseases, such as age-related macular degeneration, cataracts and dry eye syndrome.

As an optometrist by profession and a food lover by nature, I became excited early on in my career about the power of certain foods to help prevent eye disease. My passion for ocular nutrition began more than 10 years ago, after I saw the effects eye disease had on my patients' lives. I wanted to give my patients information about what they could do to help prevent eye disease and maintain their ocular health. I found myself attending conferences about ocular nutrition and reading everything I could about the relationship of nutrients and food to eye health and function. As I immersed myself in the research, a light bulb went off in my head and I realized that nutritional guidance was what was missing from my practice.

At the time, it was a standard of care to recommend certain vitamins for patients who had moderate age-related macular degeneration (AMD), to help prevent progression to advanced AMD. But my patients often asked what foods contained the same nutrients. In particular, they wanted to know if there were foods they could add to their diet, in addition to the vitamin supplements, that might help protect their eyes. I wanted to tell them more than simply "Eat spinach." I became inspired to continue increasing my knowledge about the role of nutrition in ocular health and to start talking to more of my patients about it.

I soon realized the magnitude of the project I was undertaking and knew I couldn't do it alone. At that time, my great friend and colleague Dr. Barbara Pelletier joined me in analyzing the research on ocular nutrition and determining the nutrient content of hundreds of whole foods. Together, we developed a list of foods that contain high amounts of eye-healthy nutrients. We decided to call these foods "eyefoods."

We began to incorporate eyefoods into our own families' diets and started to share this information with our patients. We quickly discovered that people did not want general knowledge; rather, they wanted a plan. They wanted to know how much of each food they needed to eat and how to integrate the foods into their diet. This feedback led us to develop the Eyefoods Plan, an easy-to-follow dietary plan that provides exactly the type of guidance our patients wanted.

Everyone will benefit from adding eyefoods to their diet. In fact, I believe so strongly that everyone should follow an eye-healthy diet and lifestyle, I share nutrition and lifestyle information with all of the patients in my practice, Eye Wellness, an innovative vision and eye health clinic that brings together optometry, nutrition and lifestyle education. I am grateful for my patients, as their curiosity and motivation to make better everyday choices for their eye health inspire me daily to continue learning about the field of ocular nutrition. I am excited to share this information with you.

In *Eyefoods*, we will explore how vision works and learn about the most common eye conditions and diseases. This will establish a foundation of knowledge about the eye and vision that will help you understand the role of nutrition and lifestyle in preventing eye disease and maintaining ocular health. And to help you integrate eyefoods into your diet, this book includes a multitude of delicious and nutritious recipes for meals that will nourish your eyes with important nutrients for eye health and function.

> Whether you have an existing eye condition or are trying to maintain healthy eyes, the recommendations in this book will help you preserve your vision.

The Evidence

The information in this book is based on scientific literature and recommendations made by reputable agencies such as the American Academy of Ophthalmology, the American Optometric Association, the Canadian Association of Optometrists, the American Heart Association, the Heart and Stroke Foundation of Canada, the American Diabetes Association and Diabetes Canada. I also make practical recommendations based on my real-life experience in treating patients during my 20 years of practice.

Part 1: Eye Health and Disease

Chapter 1, "Eye Anatomy and Vision," will help you understand how the eye works. Chapter 2, "Taking Care of Your Eyes, Decade by Decade," explores how vision evolves throughout our lifespan and provides practical information on eye health and vision in every decade of life, along with tips to help you experience your best vision in each decade.

Chapter 3, "Common Eye Conditions and Diseases," highlights the relationship between nutrition and the most common eye conditions and diseases: age-related macular degeneration, cataracts, dry eye syndrome, eyelid disorders and glaucoma, as well as ocular effects related to diabetes.

Part 2: The Eyefoods Plan

Keep this book handy and browse through it frequently. You may learn something new each time you pick it up.

After a careful review of scientific studies, Dr. Pelletier and I determined the most important nutrients for the prevention of eye disease and promotion of eye health. Each of these nutrients helps to decrease the risk for eye disease, either on its own or in conjunction with other nutrients. In chapter 4, "Eye Nutrients," you will learn where these nutrients can be found in the eye and how they can help to maintain eye health.

Dr. Pelletier and I carefully analyzed hundreds of whole foods to learn which ones contain the most eye nutrients. Chapter 5, "Eyefoods," describes the foods we have included in our list of eyefoods, explores their nutritional benefits and discusses how these benefits relate to eye health. It also includes recommendations on how much of each food to include in your diet and tips on preparation.

In addition to nutrition, other important lifestyle factors, such as smoking, exercise, ultraviolet light and technology use, can affect your eye health and vision. Chapter 6, "Lifestyle and General Health," provides advice that will help you lead an eye-healthy lifestyle. You'll learn how to protect your eyes from UV light and choose the best sunglasses, strategies for protecting your eyes while using computers or devices, and information on quitting smoking, maintaining a healthy body weight and being active.

Chapter 7, "Following the Eyefoods Plan," helps you put all of this information together and outlines an easy-to-follow plan for incorporating eyefoods into your everyday life. Chapter 8, "Integrating Eyefoods into Your Diet," provides 2 weeks of sample meal plans, with shopping lists, to help you get started.

Part 3: Recipes for Healthy Eyes

While educating yourself about the best nutrients and foods for ocular health is important, including these foods in your everyday diet is the key to maintaining your best possible eye health. Part 3 includes more than 100 recipes, covering every meal of the day. Most of them are very easy to make and include a variety of eyefoods, such as green and orange vegetables and fruits. Smoothies and salads, for example, are both great ways to enjoy fruits and vegetables with very little work.

Scattered throughout the book, you'll find interesting facts and tips about eyefoods and eye health. I am excited to share this book with you and hope to inspire you to make everyday choices that may lead you to a lifetime of healthier eyes.

PART 1

Eye Health and Disease

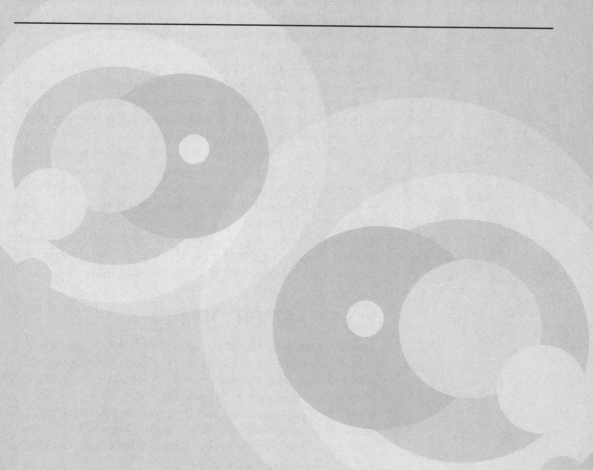

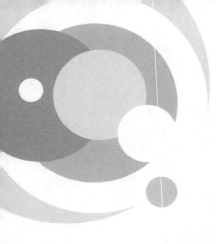

Chapter 1

Eye Anatomy and Vision

The risk of many eye diseases can be decreased with a healthy diet and lifestyle — you hold the keys to your eye health.

During my years of optometric practice, I have found that most people consider vision to be one of their most important senses. Maintaining healthy eyes is a priority for everyone, and my patients frequently ask how they can keep their eyes strong and preserve their vision. Current research has taught us that the risk of many eye diseases can be decreased with a healthy diet and lifestyle — you hold the keys to your eye health.

The first step in preserving your vision or dealing with an existing eye condition is to educate yourself about eye health and eye disease. Many people wear corrective lenses — glasses or contact lenses — to see better at a distance, for reading or both. Most people who wear corrective lenses do not have eye disease, but rather something called refractive error. If you have a refractive error and healthy eyes, you should be able to achieve 20/20 vision when you wear glasses or contact lenses.

Common eye conditions include cataracts, age-related macular degeneration, dry eye syndrome, glaucoma and diabetic retinopathy. An eye condition can affect the clarity of your vision or the comfort and appearance of your eyes. For example, dry eye syndrome can occasionally cause fluctuating vision, but it more commonly causes foreign body sensation (feeling like something is in your eye), dry eyes or watery eyes.

Knowing how the eye works will help you understand how nutrition and lifestyle contribute to eye health. This chapter explains the important structures of the eye, explores the visual process and reviews which eye conditions affect each structure. It also highlights the nutrients that are most important for healthy eye function and illustrates where these nutrients can be found in the eye.

Eye Anatomy

To understand how and why nutrition and lifestyle play a role in maintaining the health of our eyes, it helps to learn about the anatomy of the eye. The eye is made up of two parts: the anterior (front) segment, which includes the tear film, sclera, conjunctiva, cornea, iris, pupil and lens; and the posterior (back) segment, which includes the vitreous humor, retina, macula, fovea and optic nerve. Each part of the eye serves an important function in vision and maintaining healthy eyes.

FAQ

Q. How often should I have an eye examination?

A. Regular eye examinations by an optometrist or ophthalmologist are important for early diagnosis and treatment of eye conditions. Even if you have never had any vision problems, regular eye examinations will help prevent vision loss from eye disease. An optometrist or ophthalmologist can diagnose many eye diseases that do not have noticeable symptoms.

After your first comprehensive eye examination, your eye doctor will determine if more frequent eye examinations are necessary.

The American Optometric Association and Canadian Association of Optometrists recommend the following guidelines for eye examinations for people who are at low risk for developing eye problems.

Age Group	Minimum Recommended Frequency of Eye Examination
Infants and toddlers (birth to 24 months)	By age 6 months
Preschool children (2 to 5 years)	At age 3
School-age (6 to 17 years)	Before first grade and annually thereafter
Adults (18 to 60 years)	Every 1 to 2 years
Older adults (61 years and older)	Annually

Sources: American Optometric Association: www.aoa.org/patients-and-public/caring-for-your-vision/comprehensive-eye-and-vision-examination/recommended-examination-frequency-for-pediatric-patients-and-adults; Canadian Association of Optometrists: opto.ca/health-library/frequency-of-eye-examinations.

Tear Film

The tear film is the outermost layer of the eye. It provides stability to our vision and lubricates the underlying structures (the conjunctiva and cornea). Our tears are made up of three main components: the lipid (or oil) layer, the aqueous (or watery) layer and the mucin (or mucus) layer. Dry eye syndrome affects the tear film.

Sclera

The sclera is the outermost white part of the eye. It protects the eyeball and is made up of collagen. The sclera and cornea are both outer surfaces of the eye. They are joined by the limbus.

Conjunctiva

The conjunctiva is the mucous membrane that covers the outer surface of the eye. The bulbar conjunctiva covers the sclera, and the palpebral conjunctiva covers the inside of the eyelids. The bulbar conjunctiva is covered with the tear film. It keeps the front of the eye lubricated and protects the eye from dust and debris.

DID YOU KNOW?

The Eye Is Not a Perfect Sphere

Although the "eyeball" is round, it is not a perfect sphere, because the cornea, which is the clear outer tissue of the eye, has a different curvature than the sclera, which is the outer white part of the eye.

Cornea

The cornea is the clear outer tissue of the eye. It is the first surface to refract, or bend, light to focus on the retina. For optimal vision, it is important that the corneal tissue be clear. Scarring of the cornea can distort or blur vision. Dry eye syndrome can cause inflammation of the cornea or corneal staining.

Iris

The iris is the colored part of the eye. It controls the amount of light that enters the eye by opening and closing the pupil.

Pupil

The pupil is the dark opening at the center of the iris. It is actually a hole that changes size depending on lighting conditions. In bright light, the pupil is small. In darkness, the pupil is larger, to allow more light into the eye.

Lens

The lens is located behind the iris. Both the lens and the cornea refract light to focus on the retina. The clarity of the lens is important for clear vision. A cataract is a cloudiness of the lens and may cause gradual blurry vision.

Aqueous Humor

The aqueous humor is located in the anterior chamber (in the area between the cornea and iris) and in the posterior chamber (in the area between the lens and the retina). It keeps the eyeball inflated and maintains intraocular pressure. It also provides nutrition to the cornea and lens.

Choroid

The choroid is the tissue between the sclera and the retina. It is a vascular tissue, containing blood vessels and connective tissue. The choroid provides nourishment to the retina. In diseases such as wet age-related macular degeneration (see page 30), blood from the choroid can migrate to the retina and cause loss or distortion of vision.

Vitreous Humor

The vitreous humor is located in the posterior chamber of the eye, and looks and feels like jelly. It is transparent, which means it allows light to pass through it. The vitreous is made up of water, collagen fibers and hyaluronic acid. As we age, it can liquefy or develop a change in consistency that can cause floaters. Floaters have different shapes and sizes, but usually appear as spots, threads or cobwebs in a person's vision.

Retina

The retina is a sensory membrane at the back of the eye. Its main purpose is to convert light into electrical impulses that are transmitted to the brain by way of the optic nerve. Rods and cones are cells in the retina that are also known as photoreceptors. They are light-sensitive cells that initiate the vision signal. Rods work in dim light and are responsible for detecting motion and for black-and-white vision. Cones work in bright light and are responsible for fine-detailed central vision and color vision. Diabetic retinopathy is a condition that affects the retina.

Macula and Fovea

The macula, located in the center of the retina, allows for fine visual acuity and central vision. It allows us to see details, to read and to see faces. The fovea is located in the center of the macula and is the point of maximal visual acuity. The only photoreceptors in the fovea are cones. Age-related macular degeneration and diabetic macular edema are diseases that affect the macula.

Optic Nerve

The optic nerve is the second cranial nerve (see sidebar). It originates at the back of the eye and travels through the brain to the occipital cortex, transmitting visual information.

(see sidebar)

DID YOU KNOW?

Cranial Nerves

Cranial nerves carry information from the brain to various parts of the body. There are 12 cranial nerves, numbered in order of the position from which they exit the brain and lead into the body, from front to back. The first cranial nerve is the olfactory nerve, which is responsible for our sense of smell. The second is the optic nerve.

The Parts of the Eye

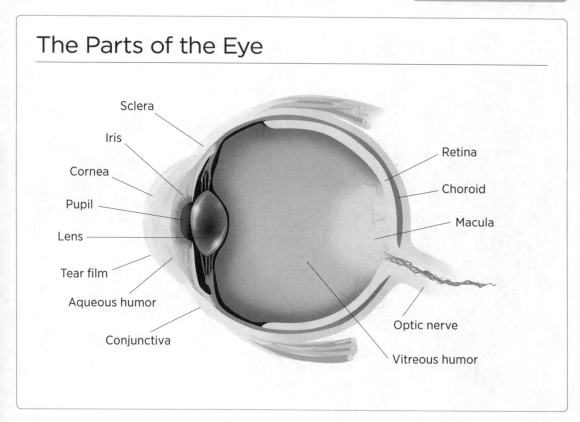

Sclera
Iris
Cornea
Pupil
Lens
Tear film
Aqueous humor
Conjunctiva
Retina
Choroid
Macula
Optic nerve
Vitreous humor

The Visual Process

We usually attribute our vision to our eyes; however, the brain plays an important role in vision. Essentially, we need both our eyes and our brain to see. Here is a step-by-step guide to the visual process:

1. Light bounces off an object the eye is looking at.
2. This light passes through the cornea. The pupil changes size to adjust to how much light is coming in. In darkness, the pupil dilates (gets larger); in brightness, it constricts.
3. The light then passes through the lens. Both the cornea and the lens are curved, so the light refracts (bends) as it passes through. This helps it focus on a specific point on the retina. The lens inverts the image so that it is upside down when it reaches the retina.
4. Light focuses at the macula, and the macula creates the vision signal.
5. The vision signal passes through the optic nerve to the visual cortex.
6. The visual cortex in the occipital lobe of the brain processes vision. The information is received upside down, and the visual cortex flips it right-side up.

The Visual Process

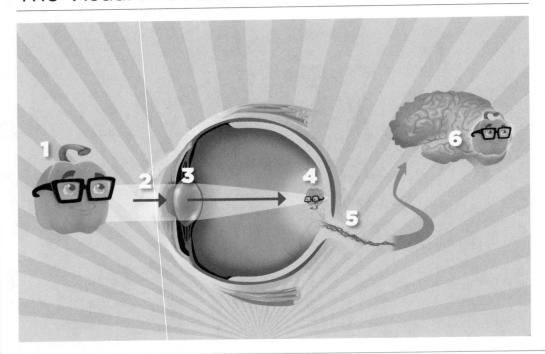

Refractive Errors

A refractive error is not a problem with ocular health; rather, it is an issue with focusing light. People with "normal vision" are emmetropic, meaning that the images they see are focused directly on the macula when their eyes are in a relaxed state. People who are emmetropic do not have a refractive error and do not require glasses or contact lenses to correct their vision.

Refractive errors include myopia, hyperopia, astigmatism and presbyopia, and it is possible to have a combination of different refractive errors. People with one or more refractive errors may require glasses or contact lenses to help them see clearly.

Myopia (Nearsightedness)

The light entering the eye focuses in front of the macula, resulting in blurry distance vision. Myopia often occurs when the length of the eyeball from the cornea to the retina is too long, or when the cornea and/or the lens are too steep to focus the light on the retina. (A steep cornea or lens is more curved and bends the light too much, so that it becomes focused too soon in the eye, before it reaches the retina.) Myopia can be corrected with glasses, contact lenses or laser surgery.

Hyperopia (Farsightedness)

The light entering the eye focuses beyond the macula, resulting in blurrier vision close up than at a distance. Hyperopia occurs when the eyeball is too short, or the cornea or lens is not steep enough to focus the light on the retina. It can be corrected with glasses, contact lenses or laser surgery.

Astigmatism

Like myopia and hyperopia, astigmatism is a refractive error that can be corrected with glasses, contact lenses or laser surgery. With astigmatism, the prescription in one direction is different from the prescription 90 degrees away. Astigmatism is often caused by irregularities in the shape of the cornea or lens. Small amounts of astigmatism are quite common. In fact, most glasses prescriptions include a correction for astigmatism.

Presbyopia

The age-related loss of focusing ability up close, presbyopia usually becomes noticeable between the ages of 40 and 45. You will notice the first symptoms of presbyopia when you start to hold books or your devices farther away from your face. When presbyopia occurs, the prescription you require to see in the distance is different from what you need for up close.

Presbyopia is corrected by reading glasses, which allow you to see close things clearly but make your distance vision blurry, or by progressive glasses, which allow you to see clearly at all distances by looking through different parts of the lens. Multifocal contact lenses and laser surgery can also correct presbyopia in some people.

Eye Nutrition Basics

In chapter 4, we will explore in detail how certain nutrients can help decrease the risk of eye diseases such as cataracts and macular degeneration. Numerous scientific studies have shown that foods that contain antioxidants and omega-3 fatty acids are beneficial to eye health. A diet that focuses on prevention of ocular disease will include foods that are high in beta-carotene, lutein, zeaxanthin, vitamin C, vitamin E, zinc and the omega-3 fatty acids DHA and EPA.

But these "eye nutrients" do more than just prevent ocular disease. They also help the eyes function and create vision. The table on page 15 shows which parts of the eye use each of the important eye nutrients and what foods provide these nutrients.

FAQ

Q. What are the benefits of having regular eye exams?

A. Seventy-five percent of vision loss is treatable or preventable. A comprehensive regular eye examination by an optometrist (a doctor of optometry) will help diagnose, treat and prevent diseases and disorders of the eye and visual system.

During the eye examination, various tests are performed to check your vision and how your eyes work together (binocular vision). Your optometrist will also ask about your lifestyle and how you use your eyes, to determine the best solutions for you to achieve your optimal vision. They will educate you about the latest technology in vision correction, such as digital high-definition eyeglass lenses, coatings that filter blue light and minimize glare, contact lenses and refractive surgery.

In addition to checking your vision, your optometrist will evaluate your eye health. Many eye diseases, such as dry eye syndrome, glaucoma, age-related macular degeneration and diabetic retinopathy, can exist without any symptoms and must be diagnosed during an eye examination. Early diagnosis can lead to better treatment and less risk of vision loss.

A comprehensive eye examination may also include advanced testing, such as digital retinal photographs and ocular coherence tomography (OCT). These images allow the doctor to detect eye disease at the earliest onset.

Some general health conditions can also be detected through an eye examination. The health of your eyes is connected to the health of your entire body. Many doctors of optometry will address the eye–body connection and offer you a plan on how to prevent eye disease through nutrition and lifestyle.

Important Nutrients for Ocular Function and Vision

Nutrient	Location in the Eye	Foods That Contain It
Beta-carotene	Retina (the body makes vitamin A from beta-carotene; both can be found in the retina)	Carrots, sweet potatoes, winter squash
Lutein	Macula, lens	Broccoli, egg yolks, leafy greens
Omega-3 fatty acids (DHA and EPA)	Retina, Meibomian glands	Rainbow trout, salmon, sardines, tuna
Vitamin C	Cornea, aqueous humor, vitreous humor, retina, lens	Bell peppers, broccoli, citrus fruit, kiwifruit
Vitamin E	Retina	Eggs, kiwifruit, olive oil, orange bell peppers, nuts, seeds
Zeaxanthin	Macula, lens	Orange bell peppers, goji berries
Zinc	Retina (zinc is important to the function of the cells in the eye; it also transports vitamins A and E from the liver to the eye)	Oysters, turkey, red meat, nuts, whole grains

Where in the Eye Is That?

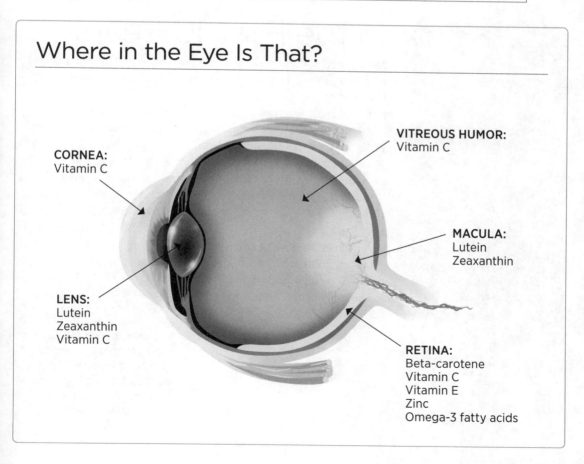

CORNEA:
Vitamin C

VITREOUS HUMOR:
Vitamin C

MACULA:
Lutein
Zeaxanthin

LENS:
Lutein
Zeaxanthin
Vitamin C

RETINA:
Beta-carotene
Vitamin C
Vitamin E
Zinc
Omega-3 fatty acids

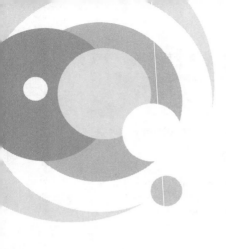

Chapter 2

Taking Care of Your Eyes, Decade by Decade

Just like our bodies, our eyes require different care at different stages of our life. In this chapter, we will look at how our eyes and vision evolve throughout each decade of life. I will note the important changes in the eyes and how we see, and highlight specific nutrients that help us maintain healthy eyes at each stage. I will also provide tips to help you experience clear vision in each decade.

In the First 10 Years

Most parents wonder what their baby can see at different stages of development. The first few years of life are a very important time in the development of a child's eyes and vision. In fact, much of the development occurs within the first 6 months of life. Knowing the milestones helps parents stimulate their baby's vision during this important time.

As babies become toddlers and preschoolers, and preschoolers grow into school-age children, their vision and visual perception continues to develop. During these years, a child's nutrition is important to their entire body's development, and especially that of their eyes. Lifestyle habits, such as wearing sun protection, also become important. If you help your child establish good eating and lifestyle habits, you will be laying a solid foundation in the early years of their life for their future health.

> **DID YOU KNOW?**
>
> **Eye Color**
>
> Babies are born with varying degrees of blue eyes. Between birth and 6 months, a pigment called melanin is deposited in the baby's iris, often changing the color from blue to shades of hazel, green, brown or gray. The amount of melanin determines the final color. If only a small amount of melanin is deposited in the iris, the eyes will remain blue.

> **Pro Tip**
>
> Breast milk is high in DHA (docosahexaenoic acid), an omega-3 fatty acid that is necessary for infant brain and eye development.

Birth to 12 Months

Frequency of Eye Exams
An infant's first eye examination should be around
6 months of age.

As much as our bodies grow from infancy to adulthood, it's
amazing to know that a baby's eye is 65% of its adult size at
birth. During the first 6 months of life, a baby goes from seeing
black-and-white outlines, with uncoordinated eye movements,
to full color differentiation and depth perception. With this in
mind, it makes sense that an infant's first eye examination should
be at around 6 months of age.

Visual Development from Birth to 12 Months

Birth	• Baby can see bright lights, black-and-white outlines and the edges of objects and faces. • Main focus is at 8–10 inches (20–25 cm) from the baby's face.
3 months	• Parent and baby can make eye contact. • Primary colors are stimulating. • Eyes can follow moving objects.
6–12 months	• Visual acuity has improved greatly (to 20/25). • Color vision may be fully developed. • Depth perception begins to develop. • The ability to focus begins to develop. • Eyes are working together (binocular vision). • Crawling encourages the development of hand-eye coordination.

What You Can Do to Stimulate Your Baby's Vision

0–3 months	• Keep a nightlight in the baby's room. • Hold toys 8–10 inches (20–25 cm) from your baby's face.
3–6 months	• Talk to your baby as you walk around the room. • Change the position of the baby's crib and the position of the baby in the crib to alter their visual stimuli. • Place a mobile above the crib.
6–12 months	• Encourage playing on the floor, especially tummy time. • Play with blocks and play hide-and-seek with your child to encourage visual memory. • Name objects to encourage visual recognition and vocabulary skills. • Encourage crawling to help hand-eye coordination develop.

Eyefoods for Preschoolers

- Make smoothies with berries, banana and spinach, for a delicious lutein-loaded treat.
- Have some fun! Make an omelet and create a face by adding orange bell pepper slices as the eyes, nose and mouth. Sauté baby spinach to add as hair.

Simple Eyefood Snacks for Kids and Teens

- A bowl of slightly thawed frozen peas
- Orange bell pepper slices with hummus
- Carrot sticks with cashew butter

Preschoolers

Frequency of Eye Exams
Children should have their eyes examined at age 3 and before entering elementary school.

Children are very active during their preschool years, and their hand-eye coordination and fine visual motor skills continue to develop during this time. Because this is such a crucial time of learning for children, it is important to make sure that their eyes are functioning properly, that they are seeing appropriately without glasses and that their eyes are working together.

The habits a child forms during these years will also shape their future. For this reason, it is important that preschoolers eat healthy foods such as fruits and vegetables, eggs and fish. Preschoolers should also be encouraged to wear sunglasses. Long-term exposure to ultraviolet (UV) light causes damage to the retina and leads to retinal disease and cataracts later in life.

Broccoli, peppers, leafy greens, citrus fruits, berries and kiwifruit are great veggie and fruit choices. Eggs are also a good food choice for preschoolers, as they contain lutein, which is important for retinal health. These foods will encourage healthy development of their bodies and eyes, and getting them used to eating healthy foods now will give them a good foundation for healthy eating habits later in life.

Elementary-Schoolers

Frequency of Eye Exams
During elementary school, children should have their eyes examined every year.

This is a common time for refractive error to develop. In other words, children may need their first pair of glasses at some point during elementary school. It is also important to ensure that your child's eyes are working together properly, and especially to detect problems with convergence (the inward turning of the eyes). If a child has problems converging their eyes, they may have difficulty reading.

Tweens and Teens

In these years, children and teens are learning the fundamentals on which they will build their knowledge and develop skills to help them prepare for the future. For this reason, it is extremely important to make sure they are seeing their best. Children sometimes don't realize that their vision is blurry — they perceive what they are seeing as normal. Other times, difficulty learning to read or trouble in school can stem from eyestrain or headaches that may occur when their eyes aren't working together or focusing properly.

Follow these steps to ensure that your child is seeing, looking and feeling their best.

Seeing Their Best

- Schedule yearly eye examinations. If your child or teen has any changes in their vision throughout the year, notify their eye doctor. Another visit may be necessary.

- If your child has been prescribed glasses, ensure that they are wearing them as directed by their eye doctor.

- Consider contact lenses. Disposable or frequent-replacement contact lenses are a great option for tweens and teens. Make sure their contact lenses are prescribed by their eye doctor. Proper fit, training and follow-up appointments are necessary to prevent eye infections and keep their eyes healthy when wearing contact lenses.

- Make sure they are seeing their best for sports. If your child wears glasses, they should wear safety glasses or contact lenses when they play sports, to avoid injury.

Looking and Feeling Their Best

- Red, itchy or watery eyes can be signs of allergies. Many children and teens suffer from allergies. Consult an eye doctor for the best prescription eye drops.

- Use artificial tears as needed for dry eyes or if your child or teen gets something in their eye.

Taking Care of Their Eyes

- Feed your child brightly colored fruits and vegetables, especially green and orange vegetables.

- Encourage your child to try new foods — more than once. It can take many tries to develop a taste for certain foods.

- Include cold-water fish, such as salmon and light tuna, in their diet. The omega-3 fatty acids in fish will help to prevent eye disease later in life and will also keep their eyes feeling great now.

DID YOU KNOW?

Omega-3s

Omega-3 fatty acids, especially DHA, are often overlooked in a child's diet. DHA is important in the development of the optic nerve and the brain. Feeding your child cold-water fish, such as salmon, rainbow trout and light tuna, will help them get adequate amounts of DHA. Yogurt and eggs that are enriched with omega-3 fatty acids are also sources of DHA, but do not contain as much DHA as cold-water fish.

Pro Tip

Eyefoods for lunch: a tuna or salmon salad sandwich on whole-grain bread is a great source of omega-3s.

In Your 20s and 30s

For work and play, this is a time of life when your vision can elevate your performance. During these years, most people can achieve a best vision of 20/20 or better, even in poor lighting conditions. While refractive error is usually stable during these years, the varying tasks we perform, such as spending hours working on computers, can pose challenges to our vision.

Seeing Your Best

- Visit your optometrist every 1 to 2 years for a complete eye examination, even if you don't wear glasses.
- If you need glasses or contact lenses, even for a slight prescription, wear them to prevent eyestrain.
- Glasses with an anti-glare coating will sharpen your vision for night driving. Glasses with a blue light filter will sharpen your vision when you're driving at night and also when you're working on a computer.
- Laser eye surgery may be an option to reduce or eliminate your need for glasses or contact lenses.
- Wear good-quality sunglasses with a UV 400 coating and a blue light filter to protect your eyes from the harmful rays of the sun.
- For enhanced vision and to decrease glare, especially if you play sports or spend time on a boat, try polarized sunglasses with anti-glare on the back surface of the lens.

Looking and Feeling Your Best

Everyone wants the bright-eyed look of the models in the fashion magazines. Their eyes are gleaming white, large and bright. However, this often isn't the natural look of our eyes. The white part of the eye — the conjunctiva — contains many small blood vessels that are necessary to nourish the eye. Our eyes look red when these blood vessels become inflamed. The key to keeping our eyes white and bright, and feeling great as a result, is to eliminate inflammation.

These tips will help your eyes look and feel their best.

- Use high-quality, preservative-free artificial teardrops to avoid dry eye, especially when working on a computer or spending time outdoors.
- If you suffer from allergies, talk to your eye doctor about prescription eye drops to reduce the symptoms of itchy, watery and red eyes.

DID YOU KNOW?

Polarized Sunglasses

Polarized sunglasses act as a "horizontal blind," letting light into your eyes from only one direction. This eliminates glare and allows you to see the world more clearly.

Pro Tip

The omega-3 fatty acids DHA and EPA help prevent dry eye syndrome and eyelid disorders that can occur due to extensive computer use or environmental factors.

- Wear sunglasses that filter UV and blue light to reduce your risk for dry eye and for pinguecula and pterygium (blister-like conditions of the eye).
- Good-quality sunglasses will help prevent wrinkles and skin cancer around the eye.
- Choose glasses and sunglasses that make you feel and look great. The more you love your glasses, the more you'll wear them.

Taking Care of Your Eyes

We often live life in the moment in our 20s and 30s, not thinking about the possibility of developing diseases when we are older. However, this is the time to take care of your eyes for the future. Spend time learning your family history and make prevention an important part of your life.

- Find out if you have a family history of age-related macular degeneration or glaucoma. Both of these diseases have a genetic risk factor.
- Know your risk factors for eye disease in addition to family history. Ask your optometrist if you are at risk for any eye disease.
- Live healthy. Maintain a healthy weight, don't smoke, and be physically active. These lifestyle habits will help you prevent chronic diseases such as age-related macular degeneration and cataracts, as well as high blood pressure (hypertension) and diabetes.

In Your 40s and 50s

Most people who have celebrated their 50th birthday can remember the day they realized that their arms were too short. Presbyopia, the loss of focusing ability, is inevitable for most of us. Some nearsighted people will retain their ability to read without glasses beyond their mid-40s, although they will have difficulty reading while wearing glasses that correct their distance vision. It's the need for reading glasses that often brings patients into my office for an eye exam.

Seeing Your Best

- Visit your optometrist every 1 to 2 years for a complete eye examination, even if you think your vision is normal.
- Ask your eye doctor about the best glasses to correct your vision. Consider single-vision reading glasses, enhanced single-vision glasses or progressive lenses (where different parts of the lens correct for different distances). Ask about the latest designs of progressive lenses.

Eyefoods Tips: In Your 20s and 30s

- Add more omega-3 fatty acids to your diet by eating cold-water fish, such as salmon, rainbow trout, sardines or light tuna. If you don't regularly eat fish, consider taking omega-3 (fish oil) supplements.
- Make sure you're eating enough fruits and veggies.
- Have a green smoothie every day (see recipes on pages 138–145).
- Eat a salad most days. Bring a mason jar salad (see recipe, page 152) for lunch.

- Special computer glasses will provide more comfortable, clearer vision and help you to maintain proper posture when using a computer, thus reducing neck problems.
- Consider multifocal or monovision contact lenses. Multifocal contacts have several different prescriptions in each lens, while monovision contacts correct one eye for distance and the other for near vision.
- Learn about refractive surgery to treat presbyopia, such as laser blended vision.
- If you have any difficulty seeing while driving at night, you may need glasses with an anti-glare coating.
- Wear good-quality sunglasses with a UV 400 coating and a blue light filter to protect your eyes from the harmful rays of the sun.
- For sports, especially water sports, consider polarized sunglasses with anti-glare coating on the back surface of the lens.
- Have one pair of sunglasses with a darker tint for extremely bright days and another pair to enhance your vision on dull days. UV light is present even on cloudy days.

Looking and Feeling Your Best

These two decades are a busy time for most of us. Our careers are often at their peak, we're taking care of our families — sometimes both our children and our parents — and we still want to have an active social life, enjoying sports and other social activities. All this busyness takes a toll on our bodies and even on the appearance of our eyes. How can we keep our eyes looking and feeling their best?

- Get your zzzs. No amount of artificial teardrops can replace 8 hours of good-quality sleep in keeping the eyes refreshed.
- Use high-quality, preservative-free artificial teardrops to keep the eyes lubricated. Common causes for dry eye are computer use, medications and menopause.
- You can develop allergies at any age. If you suffer from itchy, watery eyes, you may need eye drops for allergies. Ask your eye doctor about the best prescription eye drops.
- Avoid eye drops that claim to "take the red out." These drops contain ingredients that will cause the blood vessels in your eyes to constrict, which will offer short-term benefits but will lead to chronic red eyes in the long term.
- Hydrate. Drink eight glasses of water per day and limit your salt intake. This will reduce any puffiness under your eyelids.

- Wear good-quality sunglasses. UV rays can cause premature aging, wrinkles and skin cancer around the eye.
- Ask your eye care professional to help you choose glasses and sunglasses frames that make you look and feel great.

Taking Care of Your Eyes

- Get checked for glaucoma. This silent eye disease has no symptoms in the early stages, and early diagnosis and treatment can save your vision.
- Take care of your body. Conditions such as high blood pressure (hypertension), diabetes and autoimmune disorders can cause collateral damage to your eyes.
- Live healthy. Maintain a healthy weight, don't smoke, and be physically active. These lifestyle habits will help you prevent chronic diseases such as age-related macular degeneration and cataracts, as well as high blood pressure and diabetes.
- Focus on prevention. Stay informed, learn, read and gather information. Take steps to prevent eye diseases that are common with aging. Things change rapidly in the field of eye care. Staying up-to-date with current information from reliable sources will help you make better decisions about your health.

In Your 60s and 70s

You can't quite pinpoint it, but your vision is not as clear as it used to be. Driving at night has become more of a chore than a joy. Reading for long periods is no longer quite as enjoyable.

These complaints are quite common from patients in their 60s and 70s. During these decades, our eyes undergo changes as a result of oxidative stress caused by the environment and our diet. Cataracts, dry eye syndrome and other changes to the eye can all contribute to a decrease in overall vision, and particularly vision in low-contrast settings.

Although it's impossible to stop the natural aging process of our eyes, an eye-friendly diet and lifestyle can help you maintain the best vision possible.

Seeing Your Best

- Make sure your glasses are up-to-date. A proper prescription will help with your night driving, reading and computer vision.
- Learn about the different types of bifocal and progressive (no-line) glasses. New lens technology provides crisper, clearer vision.

Eyefoods Tips: In Your 40s and 50s

- Important eyefoods in your 40s and 50s include cold-water fish (two to three times a week), to help prevent symptoms of dry eye, and leafy green vegetables, including kale, spinach and romaine lettuce, every day. Orange bell peppers and eggs should also be staples in your diet.
- Cook rainbow trout or salmon in parchment packets weekly (see recipe, page 203). Make enough for two meals and enjoy leftovers with a green salad for lunch the next day.
- Enjoy a smoothie every day for breakfast on your way to work. (See recipes, page 138–149.)

Pro Tip

Visit your optometrist at least once a year. You may require more frequent eye exams if you have cataracts, age-related macular degeneration, glaucoma or another eye condition.

- Have a separate pair of glasses for reading or computer use. They will provide you with clearer, more comfortable vision and help you avoid neck strain.

- Consider adding an anti-glare coating to your glasses to improve your vision for driving and a blue light filter to improve your vision when using a computer.

- To protect your eyes and sharpen your vision, wear good-quality sunglasses that have UV 400 protection and a blue light filter. The lens color is your choice. Try on different colors to see which you prefer. Some people like brown tints, while others prefer gray or green.

- If you need cataract surgery, ask your surgeon about the best options for intraocular lens implants. Different implants provide different vision benefits.

- Keep your eyes lubricated. Many people don't realize that dry eye is a common cause of blurry vision.

Looking and Feeling Your Best

Do you often feel like there is something in your eye? Do your eyes water a lot? Or burn? These are all symptoms of dry eye syndrome. Dry eye is a very common condition. Most people will have dry eye at some point during their 60s and 70s. But don't worry: here are some great tips to keep your eyes feeling fresh and vibrant.

- Use high-quality, preservative-free artificial teardrops on a regular basis. Many people who have dry eye syndrome need to use artificial tears at least four times per day.

- Artificial tears are available over the counter, but be sure to use a brand recommended by your eye doctor.

- Eat foods that are high in omega-3 fatty acids, especially fish, often.

- Consider taking an omega-3 fatty acid supplement.

- Use a warm compress. The best type is an eye mask that provides moist heat at a consistent temperature for at least 10 minutes. Ask your eye doctor to recommend an eye mask for you. Most of these masks are heated in the microwave.

Eyefoods Tips: In Your 60s and 70s

- Foods high in lutein, zeaxanthin, vitamin C and omega-3 fatty acids may help to decrease the risk and progression of cataracts.

- Plant a garden and grow your own kale, bell peppers, green beans and spinach.

- Shop at your local farmers' market for fresh fruit and vegetables in season.

- Enjoy dinners of grilled or baked salmon or rainbow trout with a side of steamed green veggies, such as broccoli, green beans or peas.

Taking Care of Your Eyes

Throughout life, our bodies are exposed to many environmental stresses and toxins. Light allows us to see, but when it comes from the sun and contains UV and blue light, it can damage our eyes. Indeed, it is one of the stresses that can lead to certain eye diseases, such as cataracts and age-related macular degeneration (AMD). Here's how you can your reduce your risk for these conditions:

- Ask your eye doctor if you are developing cataracts. Most people develop cataracts in their 60s or 70s.
- Fill your diet with eyefoods to promote eye health, whether you have eye disease or not.
- If you have AMD, take an eye vitamin as recommended by your eye doctor.
- If you have a family history of AMD, ask your eye doctor whether a supplement is recommended for you.
- Exercise. Regular physical activity will keep you feeling good, reduce your risk for heart disease and, most importantly for your eyes, help protect your eyes from AMD.
- Your sunglasses should filter both UV and blue light. Buy sunglasses from an eye care professional to ensure that their quality is good. They will help prevent the progression of cataracts and AMD, and also keep you seeing better.

In Your 80s, 90s and Beyond

Everyone has a different level of vision at this stage of life. Some people maintain clear vision in both eyes, others have vision loss in one eye, and many people have low vision in both eyes, to varying degrees. While your vision will never again be as sharp and crisp as it was many years ago, there are tips, lenses and devices that can help you achieve better vision than you currently have.

Seeing Your Best

- If you have even a light glasses prescription for distance, wear your glasses for driving to ensure that you have the best vision possible.
- To avoid distortions in your peripheral vision when driving, consider making your driving glasses single-vision instead of bifocals or progressive lenses. Progressives require you to look through the center of the lens to get the best distance vision.

- Let there be light. Use a good-quality desk or floor lamp when reading, and ensure that the ceiling lights are also turned on in the room. You'll be surprised how much good lighting can improve your reading vision.

- Don't be surprised if your eye doctor recommends multiple pairs of glasses. If you want to see your best, you may need different tools for different activities.

- If you can't see well to read, even with reading glasses or progressives, tell your eye doctor. You may benefit from a magnifying glass or other low-vision device. You don't need to be legally blind to use low-vision devices; magnifiers can help people with all levels of vision.

- If you have low vision or already use a magnifier, make a low-vision appointment at least once every 2 years to see if there are new devices available that may help more.

- Make sure your sunglasses block both UV and blue light. Wear a tint that gives you the sharpest vision. There are many different colors of sunglasses lenses, and everyone has their own preference.

Looking and Feeling Your Best

- Artificial teardrops are good for your eyes. Choose high-quality, preservative-free teardrops, and use them regularly to treat dry eye and keep your eyes feeling lubricated and fresh.

- Moist heat will help the Meibomian glands in your eyelids work better. Use a heated eye mask for 10 to 15 minutes, once a day, to keep your eyelids healthy.

- Run a humidifier in your house, or at least your bedroom, during the dry months of the year, to help to prevent dry eye.

- Get your omega-3s. Omega-3 fatty acids from cold-water fish will help prevent dry eye and keep your eyes feeling good.

- Consider taking an eye supplement with omega-3 fatty acids if you have dry eye syndrome. Ask your eye doctor for a specific recommendation.

Taking Care of Your Eyes

Chances are that you've had cataract surgery, and you definitely know people who have. It is one of the most common surgeries performed today and is very safe and effective. These are also the years when the risk of age-related macular degeneration (AMD) is greatest. Glaucoma and diseases of the ocular surface, such as dry eye and eyelid disorders, are also more common.

Staying informed is paramount. Here are some tips to keep your peepers the healthiest they can be.

- Have your eyes checked at least once a year. If you have cataracts or AMD, you may need more frequent eye examinations.

- Wear good-quality sunglasses with UV and blue light filters in all seasons. The UV rays in the winter are also harmful, especially if they reflect off snow.

- Take an eye vitamin. If you have AMD, your eye doctor will recommend the best vitamin for you.

- Take care of your overall health and your heart. Conditions such as diabetes and high blood pressure (hypertension) can affect the blood vessels in the retina, causing problems with your eyes.

Eyefoods Tips: In Your 80s and 90s and Beyond

- Lutein has been related to brain health and cognitive function, so it's important to consume foods high in lutein, including leafy greens, green vegetables and eggs, on a daily basis.
- If you have trouble digesting raw fruits and veggies, blend them! Make smoothies with your favorite fruits and leafy greens. You'll find smoothie recipes on pages 138–149.
- Add kale or spinach to soups. Blend them to make them easier to digest.

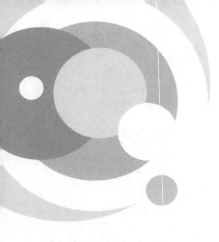

Chapter 3

Common Eye Conditions and Diseases

Remember that each person is different and that eye disease can present differently in everyone. If you think you might have an eye condition or disease, speak with your optometrist or ophthalmologist.

Learning about eye health and disease is the first step in preserving vision or dealing with an existing eye condition. It is important to differentiate a healthy eye that requires corrective lenses (glasses or contact lenses) to see clearly from an eye with a condition or disease. Most people who wear glasses or contact lenses actually have very healthy eyes and can achieve excellent vision with the help of glasses or contact lenses. And not all eye diseases or conditions cause vision loss.

Most of the diseases discussed in this chapter are related to aging or inflammation in the body. This is not a comprehensive list of all eye diseases; rather, these are the diseases that are most likely to be influenced by diet and lifestyle.

Regular Eye Examinations

The American Optometric Association recommends that adults between the ages of 18 and 61 have their eyes examined every 1 to 2 years by an optometrist or ophthalmologist, and that people over 61 have their eyes examined yearly. The Canadian Association of Optometrists recommends yearly or biannual eye exams for people between 18 and 65 and yearly exams for people over 65. Both associations recommend yearly exams for anyone who is at high risk of developing eye disease. High-risk individuals include:

- People with diabetes or high blood pressure (hypertension)
- People with a family history of ocular disease, such as glaucoma or age-related macular degeneration
- People working in occupations that are visually highly demanding or eye-hazardous
- People taking prescription or nonprescription drugs with ocular side effects
- People who wear contact lenses
- People who have had eye surgery
- People with other health concerns or conditions

Age-Related Macular Degeneration

Age-related macular degeneration (AMD) is the leading cause of vision loss in older adults (50+) in the Western world, and its effects have a great impact on people's lives and on society in general. Here are some important facts to help you understand AMD better:

- According to the U.S. National Eye Institute, the number of cases of AMD in the United States is expected to rise from 2.07 million in 2010 to 5.44 million in 2050.

- Researchers estimate that more than 2 million Canadians have some form of AMD.

- AMD is a disease of the central part of the retina — the macula — and it affects our central vision.

- AMD does not lead to total blindness, as it affects only central vision.

- The vision loss from AMD ranges from blurry and distorted central vision to complete loss of central vision, or a blind spot in the central vision.

- Many important activities for people in the high-risk age group for AMD (60+) rely on central vision. Reading, driving, using a computer and watching TV all require good central vision.

Vision Loss from AMD

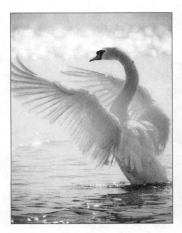

Normal vision.

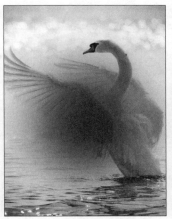

An example of the vision of a person with early AMD.

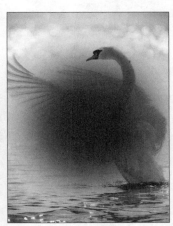

An example of the vision of a person with advanced AMD.

Dry and Wet AMD

There are two types of AMD: dry and wet. Dry AMD is the more common form, making up 85% to 90% of all AMD cases. Wet AMD is a more advanced and severe form, often causing a dramatic decrease or loss of central vision.

Neither dry AMD nor wet AMD causes total blindness; people with AMD may notice changes in their ability to read books, see street signs or see details on a person's face; however, they are able to walk and move around safely.

Dry AMD

Dry AMD occurs when the cells in the macula begin to break down, causing thinning of the macula. The retina becomes unable to rid itself of its metabolic waste, called lipofuscin. Lipofuscin accumulates in the retina as drusen, which block the normal function of the retina. Appearing in the retina as yellow spots, drusen are often the first signs of dry AMD.

Gradual central vision loss can occur with dry AMD, but in most cases, vision loss from dry AMD is less severe than from wet AMD. However, over time, changes in the retina from dry AMD can lead to a condition called geographic atrophy, which can cause severe central vision loss.

Wet AMD

In wet AMD, there is abnormal blood vessel growth in the choroid (a vascular tissue behind the retina). These blood vessels can grow into the macula through breaks in the membrane that separates the retina and the choroid, leading to rapid and dramatic vision loss caused by bleeding and leakage of the blood vessels.

Pro Tip

Dry AMD is usually a less severe form of AMD, but it can lead to wet AMD.

DID YOU KNOW?

No Help from Glasses

In most cases, AMD causes a gradual, slow loss of vision. However, vision loss can sometimes be dramatic and sudden. In either case, glasses cannot correct blurry vision, blind spots or distortions in vision caused by AMD.

Signs and Symptoms: AMD

AMD can be asymptomatic. When symptoms occur, they are related to central vision loss:

- Gradual loss of central vision
- Distortion of straight lines
- Blurry vision when reading
- Decrease in contrast sensitivity
- Rapid-onset loss of central vision
- Blind spot in or near the central vision

Risk Factors for AMD

Some of the risk factors for AMD, such as diet, lifestyle and smoking, are within our control — they are modifiable risk factors. Others, such as age and genetics, are unmodifiable.

The number one risk factor for AMD is being over 50 years old. According to the National Eye Institute, of the 2.07 million Americans with AMD in 2010, 1.32 million were over the age of 80.

Risk Factors: AMD

Unmodifiable Risk Factors

- Age (50+)
- Genetics (if you have a blood relative with AMD, your risk of developing the disease is increased)
- Sex (women are at higher risk than men)
- Eye color (light-colored eyes are at higher risk)
- Race (Caucasians are at higher risk)

Modifiable Risk Factors

- Smoking
- UV light exposure
- Blue light exposure (short-wavelength visible blue light)
- Low macular pigment (lutein, zeaxanthin and mesozeaxanthin make up the macular pigment; people with lower macular pigment have been shown to be at increased risk for AMD)
- Diets high in sugar and refined carbohydrates
- Excess weight or obesity
- Diabetes and cardiovascular disease

DID YOU KNOW?

Smoking and AMD

Scientific studies show that smoking is the most important modifiable risk factor in AMD prevention. Compared to people who have never smoked, current smokers are 45% more likely to develop early AMD or AMD progression over 15 years.

Diagnostic Tests

An optometrist or ophthalmologist can diagnose AMD during a dilated eye examination using special lenses. Other common tests that aid in the diagnosis of AMD include a thorough patient history, Amsler grid testing and imaging of the retina, including digital photography and optical coherence tomography.

Amsler Grid Testing

Symptoms of AMD progression can take the form of straight lines appearing wavy, or of blind spots appearing in your vision. An Amsler grid is a chart that can be used to monitor these possible changes in your vision.

DID YOU KNOW?

Early Diagnosis

AMD is often diagnosed during a routine eye examination, before a person has any symptoms such as blurred or distorted vision. Early diagnosis of AMD can give you the opportunity to make diet and lifestyle changes that may decrease the risk of progression of the disease.

Normal and Abnormal Amsler Grids

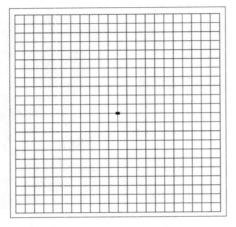

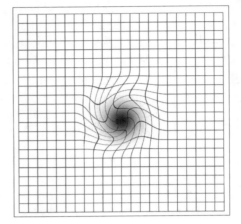

Normal vision: the grid should appear regular, with clear, straight lines.

Abnormal vision: the grid may appear distorted and/or contain blind spots. (Note: abnormalities may appear in any part of the grid.)

FAQ

Q. How do I use an Amsler grid?

A. When you look at an Amsler grid, it is important to use one eye at a time. Looking at the dot in the center of the chart, notice if any of the lines on the grid are wavy or distorted. Also observe whether there are any missing areas in the grid and ensure that you can see all four corners. If anything about how you see the grid has changed since your last appointment with your eye doctor, contact your doctor's office.

If your eye doctor has recommended that you monitor your vision with the Amsler grid, it is important to look at the grid regularly — preferably daily — as doing so will alert you to any changes in your vision in a timely manner.

Contrast Sensitivity Testing

Contrast sensitivity testing is an advanced measurement of visual function that helps to determine your vision in situations of low light, fog or glare. People with AMD will often experience a decrease in their contrast sensitivity before their visual acuity is affected. In everyday activities, this will manifest as decreased vision in low-light environments or difficulty reading fonts that are close in color to their background.

Digital Retinal Photography

A digital photograph of your retina in real time can show anatomical changes associated with AMD, and is useful for comparing changes in your retina over time.

Macular Pigment Optical Density Measurement

Low levels of macular pigment (lutein, zeaxanthin and meso-zeaxanthin) are related to a greater risk for AMD. Macular pigment optical density (MPOD) can be measured with a simple in-office test. Increasing your intake of lutein and zeaxanthin, through either diet or supplements, can improve your macular pigment levels. Repeating MPOD measurements every 6 to 12 months can determine whether the dietary changes or supplements are helping to increase your macular pigment. See chapter 4 for more information on macular pigments.

Increasing your intake of lutein and zeaxanthin, through either diet or supplements, can improve your macular pigment levels.

Fluorescein Angiography

Fluorescein angiography (FA) examines blood circulation in the retina and choroid. A fluorescent dye is injected into the patient's circulation, then a special camera is used to image the retinal blood vessels.

Optical Coherence Tomography

A leading-edge technology that uses a scanning laser to analyze the layers of the retina for signs of retinal disease, optical coherence tomography (OCT) is a noninvasive, painless test that can show early signs of AMD, especially early development of wet AMD. It is also important in monitoring the efficacy of treatment for wet AMD.

Optical Coherence Tomography Angiography

This novel technology is a noninvasive procedure that provides imaging of the blood vessels in the retina. Unlike fluorescein angiography, there is no dye injection; instead, OCT angiography uses motion of the blood cells, a technique that is much faster than fluorescein angiography. More information about the retinal blood vessels is obtained from OCT angiography than from OCT.

Genetic Testing for AMD

From a genetic standpoint, AMD is a complex disease. To date, 34 genetic loci and 54 gene variants have been identified as related to AMD risk. Genetic testing is currently available to assess AMD risk; however, the clinical use of these tests has been very controversial amongst optometrists, ophthalmologists and scientists in the eye care world. Some studies have raised questions about whether AMD may be more likely to progress with the use of standard nutritional supplements commonly recommended in AMD treatment for people with a certain genetic profile. However, other analyses contradict these findings.

Our understanding of the genetics of AMD and how it relates to other risk factors is still evolving. The question is, Will you benefit from taking a genetic test? Will the information you learn from the test help you reduce your risk of developing AMD, or reduce your risk of vision loss from AMD?

My recommendation is to discuss this with your optometrist and/or ophthalmologist. Your eye care team has your best interests in mind and will give you good advice based on the most current knowledge available. In my opinion, any type of genetic testing must be taken seriously and should be accompanied by genetic counseling. You need to be aware of how the information you receive regarding your genetic profile and risk will benefit your health.

At the time of writing, the American Academy of Ophthalmology discourages the use of routine genetic testing for AMD in the clinical setting.

Current Treatments

The goal in the treatment of dry AMD is to reduce the risk of progression and, as a result, maintain the best possible vision.

The field of research in the area of AMD is evolving at a rapid pace. At this time, there is no cure for dry AMD. The goal in the treatment of dry AMD is to reduce the risk of progression and, as a result, maintain the best possible vision. The lifestyle checklist on page 35 may help you to decrease your risk of dry AMD progression.

There are several treatment options for wet AMD, depending on the stage of the disease and the location of the abnormal blood vessels. In the past, wet AMD was treated with laser photocoagulation or photodynamic therapy with Visudyne. Current treatments include anti-VEGF (vascular endothelial growth factor) injections, which block the protein (VEGF) that is responsible for new blood vessel growth. In wet AMD, anti-VEGF injections help stop the growth of new blood vessels in the retina. They may slow the progression of vision loss and, in some cases, even improve vision. An ophthalmologist injects the medication into the eye. Multiple injections, given on a monthly basis, are often required for the treatment to be effective. Before you receive the injection, an anesthetic is instilled into the eye to minimize any discomfort.

Lifestyle Checklist for AMD

If you have risk factors for AMD, following these diet and lifestyle suggestions may decrease your risk for developing the disease. If you already have AMD, they may decrease the risk of the disease progressing and may help to minimize vision loss.

- ○ Eat foods rich in the carotenoids lutein and zeaxanthin, such as leafy greens, orange bell peppers and eggs.

- ○ Eat cold-water fish, such as salmon, rainbow trout, sardines, mackerel or light tuna, at least twice a week to enjoy the benefits of high levels of omega-3 fatty acids.

- ○ Take an eye vitamin that includes lutein and zeaxanthin, vitamin C, vitamin E and zinc. Ask your eye doctor to recommend the best supplement for you.

- ○ Engage in regular physical activity and maintain a healthy weight.

- ○ Don't smoke.

- ○ Have your eyes checked regularly. Many people with dry AMD should visit their eye doctor at least every 6 months and may benefit from retinal photography, optical coherence tomography (OCT) or macular pigment optical density (MPOD) tests.

- ○ Use an Amsler grid daily. The Amsler grid is a simple test that allows you to notice early changes of distorted vision, which may be a sign of progression of dry AMD to wet AMD.

- ○ Protect your eyes from UV and blue light by wearing good-quality sunglasses with a UV 400 coating and a blue light filter.

Pro Tip

To date, anti-VEGF medication is the only treatment that has resulted in an improvement in visual acuity.

DID YOU KNOW?

Dietary Risk Factors for AMD

- A diet high in sugar
- A diet with a high glycemic index
- Excess weight or obesity

FAQ

Q. I've been diagnosed with AMD. What should I ask my optometrist or ophthalmologist?

A. Receiving a diagnosis of AMD can leave you feeling afraid, confused and unsure about the future of your vision. Most AMD is dry AMD, which does not lead to severe loss of vision. However, it is important to know more about your diagnosis so you can make diet and lifestyle changes to help reduce the risk of progression of the disease. Here are some questions to ask your eye doctor:

- Do I have dry or wet AMD?
- How often should I use my Amsler grid?
- Do you recommend that I take supplements to help prevent progression? If so, which supplements do you recommend?
- What changes should I look for in my vision that could indicate the AMD is progressing? When should I call your office?

Research Spotlight

Controlling AMD with Diet

Numerous studies have shown a relationship between nutrition and AMD. To date, the most significant studies are the Age-Related Eye Disease Study and its follow-up study (AREDS 1 and AREDS 2). AREDS 1 was a large, randomized, controlled trial that followed more than 3,000 participants for 7 years and concluded that taking a supplement with specific antioxidants and zinc decreases the risk of progression of AMD in certain patients by as much as 25%.

The follow-up study, AREDS 2, assessed the effects of supplementing patients' diets with high doses of two carotenoids (lutein and zeaxanthin) and omega-3 fatty acids. The study concluded that adding 10 milligrams of lutein and 2 milligrams of zeaxanthin reduced the progression from dry AMD to wet AMD by 11% compared to the original AREDS formulation. The study also found that the addition of lutein and zeaxanthin reduced the progression to legal blindness by 18%. No effect on the progression of AMD was seen in the study participants with the addition of omega-3 fatty acids (350 milligrams of DHA and 650 milligrams of EPA).

Eye care professionals recommend that most patients with AMD take an AREDS-type vitamin supplement. However, a supplement is not a replacement for a healthy diet. The synergy of the nutrients in whole foods has a beneficial effect on our bodies that a supplement cannot replicate. Many other studies have found that diets high in certain nutrients help to reduce the risk of AMD, and that poor diets can increase a person's risk for developing the disease.

Visual Aids

Many people with AMD realize the effect of the disease when their vision doesn't improve with new glasses. If your glasses cannot correct your vision to be clear enough for your daily activities, you may benefit from a visual aid. With rapid changes in technology, the available options in visual aids are increasing.

Visual aids are devices that help people with low vision function by maximizing their remaining eyesight. They often involve the use of magnifiers (handheld, mounted or stand-alone), telescopes and other tools to enlarge the images of objects, making them more visible. Some visual aids reduce glare and enhance contrast, which makes it easier to see. Others act as guides to help you focus on nonvisual cues, such as sound or feel.

Finding the right visual aid is a matter of consulting with a professional to learn what technology exists to make your life simpler, and experimenting with what works for you in the context of your daily needs.

DID YOU KNOW?

Stair Safety

Adding high-contrast stripes to staircases (a bright color on dark stairs or black stripes on light-colored stairs) can help prevent falls and may enable people with low vision to remain independent in their home.

Tips to Maximize Your Vision

- Ensure that you have adequate lighting in your home. This may require some trial and error with different lights and voltages to determine the best lighting for you.

- Use a magnifier. A vast selection is available, ranging from handheld to stand magnifiers. Binoculars and spectacle-mounted magnifiers are other options.

- Ask your optometrist or low-vision specialist to recommend specialized lens tints that enhance vision or reduce light sensitivity for certain conditions, such as retinitis pigmentosa or cataracts.

- Read large-print books or try digital recordings or MP3s.

- Make use of high contrast for writing. Try writing in large letters with a broad black pen on white paper or a whiteboard.

If your glasses cannot correct your vision to be clear enough for your daily activities, you may benefit from a visual aid.

FAQ

Q. What foods can I eat to decrease my risk for AMD?

A. Studies show that eating foods high in lutein, zeaxanthin, omega-3 fatty acids, vitamin C, vitamin E and zinc can help reduce the risk of AMD. Follow these four simple tips to increase the amount of these important nutrients in your diet.

- **Leafy greens:** A handful a day helps keep AMD away. Kale, spinach, Swiss chard, rapini, dandelion greens, watercress and collard greens contain high amounts of lutein and all of the other eye-healthy nutrients. Eat them every day, enjoying them both cooked and raw to reap their full benefits.

- **Orange bell peppers:** Eat two orange peppers a week, both raw and cooked. All bell peppers are good choices for eye health, but the orange ones are particularly good. They contain high amounts of both lutein and zeaxanthin, and more vitamin C than yellow, red or green peppers.

- **Cold-water fish:** Eat three to four servings of fish per week. Wild salmon, rainbow trout, sardines, mackerel and light tuna contain high amounts of the omega-3 fatty acids DHA and EPA, and are low in contaminants.

- **Eggs:** Eat four eggs a week. Egg yolks contain a form of lutein that is absorbed very well by our bodies. Egg yolks are also a good source of vitamin E and zinc. Choose eggs fortified with omega-3 fatty acids for even more benefits.

In Summary

- Age-related macular degeneration is the leading cause of blindness in the Western world.
- AMD affects central vision only. It does not lead to total blindness.
- There are two types of AMD: dry AMD and wet AMD. Dry AMD is more common and less severe than wet AMD. In some cases, dry AMD can progress to wet AMD.
- Diets high in antioxidants, carotenoids (lutein and zeaxanthin) and omega-3 fatty acids may help to prevent AMD or reduce the risk of it progressing.
- Smoking increases the risk of AMD.
- People with signs of early to intermediate AMD are generally advised to take an AREDS-based vitamin supplement, to follow a diet filled with eyefoods and to visit their eye doctor regularly.

Cataracts

A cataract is a condition in which the lens of the eye loses its transparency. As we age, our lenses become cloudy, causing a gradual blurring of vision along with reduced night vision. Many people do not know they have cataracts because the change in their vision is so gradual.

Signs and Symptoms: Cataracts

- Reduced distance and/or near vision when wearing proper corrective lenses
- Dim or blurry vision
- Difficulty driving at night
- Experiencing glare when looking at oncoming headlights or streetlights at night
- More light required for reading
- Increased nearsightedness (a change in corrective lens prescription)

Types of Cataracts

There are three main types of cataracts: nuclear sclerosis, anterior cortical cataracts and posterior subcapsular cataracts. In most cases, a cataract presents itself as a combination of the three types.

Pro Tip

Cataracts are most common in people over the age of 60; however, certain types of cataracts can occur in younger people.

Nuclear Sclerosis

In this type of cataract, the center part of the lens, the nucleus, becomes cloudy and yellows. As a patient with this type of cataract, you will experience a gradual blurring of vision, and colors may not appear as vibrant as normal. Nuclear sclerosis is the cataract most associated with aging.

Anterior Cortical Cataracts

These cataracts appear as spoke-like cloudiness in the anterior cortex, the front part of the lens. They often cause difficulty with vision in dark conditions, particularly while driving at night.

Posterior Subcapsular Cataracts

Posterior subcapsular cataracts usually progress more quickly than other cataracts and are more likely to appear in younger people. Corticosteroid medication taken over a prolonged period can increase the risk for posterior subcapsular cataracts. People who are taking corticosteroids should have regular eye health examinations.

Risk Factors: Cataracts

- Age
- Medications (taking steroids over long periods of time increases the risk of posterior subcapsular cataracts)
- UV light exposure
- Family history (helps to predict when cataracts will develop)
- A diet excessively high in sugar and refined carbohydrates

Vision Loss from Cataracts

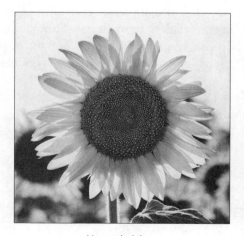

Normal vision.

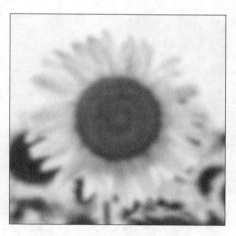

An example of the vision of a person with cataracts.

Diagnosing Cataracts

An optometrist or ophthalmologist can diagnose cataracts by using a high-powered microscope during a dilated eye examination. You may be told you have early cataracts even before you notice any changes in your vision.

Cataracts progress at different rates in different people, so it is important to talk to your eye doctor about the stage of your cataracts. If you have early signs of cataracts, you may be able to decrease their rate of progression by consuming a diet rich in omega-3 fatty acids, antioxidants and the carotenoids lutein and zeaxanthin, and by wearing sunglasses to protect your eyes from UV and blue light.

Current Treatment

Cataract surgery is the only treatment for moderate to advanced cataracts. An ophthalmologist performs surgery on patients if the cataracts are visually and clinically significant. If surgery is required, you may be given the option of either traditional cataract surgery or laser-assisted cataract surgery. With laser-assisted surgery, a laser is used to make the corneal incision and the opening in the lens capsule. The laser may also be used to soften the cataract.

In both types of surgery, ultrasound technology known as phacoemulsification is used to break up the cataract before it is removed. The surgeon then removes the lens of the eye and replaces it with an intraocular lens (IOL) implant. Many different types of IOLs are available (see below); ask your eye surgeon which is best for you.

Cataract surgery is generally a safe procedure, and the risk of complications is very low. It is usually done on an outpatient basis and doesn't require an overnight hospital stay. Most people feel no pain or discomfort during or after surgery. The surgery is performed in either a hospital or a clinic, depending on regional policies.

Recovery time after cataract surgery varies, but many people see an improvement in their vision within a few days. Most people will no longer require glasses to see at a distance, though they may still need to use reading glasses. Your surgeon or optometrist will assess your eyes at scheduled follow-up visits.

DID YOU KNOW?

Dry Eye after Cataract Surgery

Dry eye is a common side effect after any eye surgery, including cataract surgery. Burning, irritated, dry or watery eyes are some symptoms you may notice. To help prevent dry eye, it is advisable to treat it *before* cataract surgery by using high-quality, preservative-free artificial teardrops. Increasing your intake of omega-3 fatty acids, through diet or supplements, may also help you manage dry eye symptoms.

Types of Intraocular Lens Implants

- **Monofocal IOLs:** These implants offer vision correction at a specific distance to correct nearsightedness or farsightedness. For example, a patient with simple nearsightedness can have their distance vision corrected with a monofocal lens so that glasses are necessary only for near activities such as computer use, reading or doing crafts. If you have significant astigmatism, glasses may also be necessary for distance vision after cataract surgery with a monofocal IOL.

- **Toric IOLs:** These premium IOLs can correct nearsightedness, farsightedness and astigmatism. If you have significant astigmatism, a toric IOL may eliminate the need for glasses for distance vision after cataract surgery.
- **Presbyopia-correcting IOLs:** These include multifocal IOLs and accommodating IOLs. Both options offer correction of both distance and near vision. In most cases, they decrease your need for glasses for most activities. However, some patients who receive them will need glasses for night driving, reading or computer use. Not everyone is a good candidate for a presbyopic IOL, so it is important to discuss this option with your surgeon and your optometrist.

Cataract surgery is generally a safe procedure, and the risk of complications is very low.

In Summary

- A cataract is a loss of transparency in the lens of the eye.
- Cataracts are most commonly seen in people over the age of 60.
- Cataracts usually progress slowly, causing a gradual change in vision.
- Antioxidants, carotenoids (lutein and zeaxanthin) and omega-3 fatty acids may protect against the development or progression of cataracts.
- Diets with a high glycemic index have been shown to increase the risk of cataracts.
- UV light exposure increases the risk of cataracts.
- Cataract surgery, a low-risk procedure with a high success rate, is the only treatment for cataracts.
- During cataract surgery, a surgeon implants an intraocular lens into the eye, often eliminating the need for glasses.

Dry Eye Syndrome

Dry eye syndrome, also called ocular surface disease, does not necessarily mean someone has a deficiency of tears; rather, it means there is an imbalance of the tear film. It is a very common eye condition in people of all ages. Although it does not usually cause significant vision loss, as AMD and cataracts do, it does have a significant impact on overall eye health, and its symptoms can affect a person's quality of life.

The tear film is composed of three layers: aqueous (water), lipid (oil) and mucin (mucus). The lipid layer is closest to the air and is responsible for preventing evaporation of our tears. The oils in the lipid layer are produced in glands, called Meibomian glands, that run up and down in the eyelids. The aqueous layer is the middle layer of the tear film and is produced in the lachrymal glands in the upper eyelids. The mucin layer is closest to the cornea and is produced by cells in the eye called goblet cells. One of the functions of the mucin layer is to help the tear film adhere to the eye and spread evenly across the eye surface.

Various factors (see "Risk Factors for Dry Eye Syndrome," page 43) can disrupt the balance of the three layers. Each layer of our tear film plays an important role in eye health, and if any of these layers is out of balance or disrupted, you may experience dry eye syndrome.

The tear film has five main functions:

1. **Lubrication:** Tears lubricate the cornea and help maintain the health of the underlying structures. When we blink, we are continually creating friction; a healthy tear film prevents damage to the surface of the cornea and conjunctiva from that friction.

2. **Vision:** A proper tear film maintains optical stability and allows us to achieve clear vision. One of the first symptoms of dry eye is fluctuating vision, which is much like looking through a dirty windshield in a car: like a windshield wiper, with each blink, your eyelid temporarily makes things clearer.

3. **Fighting disease:** Tears have antimicrobial properties that help prevent eye infections.

4. **Corneal nutrition:** The cornea is a clear tissue that does not contain blood vessels, so tears are its main source of nutrients.

5. **Flushing debris:** Have you ever wondered why your eyes water so much when you get something in them? Tears are an automatic response to flush out any foreign body that could potentially harm the eye.

The symptoms of dry eye syndrome vary greatly. People who suffer from this condition rarely report that their eyes actually feel dry. Mild dry eye syndrome may cause the feeling that something is in the eye or a burning sensation. Moderate to severe dry eye syndrome can cause eye pain and profound watering of the eyes.

Dry eye syndrome affects people of all ages with varying degrees of severity, and its symptoms are one of the most common reasons that people seek eye care.

Signs and Symptoms: Dry Eye Syndrome

Fluctuating vision is often one of the first symptoms of dry eye. However, most people do not associate changes in their vision with dry eye and may not be motivated to seek early treatment. Other more well-known symptoms, such as burning and red eyes, appear at a more advanced stage. If you suffer from dry eye, you may experience one or many of these symptoms:

- Fluctuating vision
- Burning eyes
- Watery eyes
- Foreign body sensation (feeling like something is in your eye)

- Redness
- Discharge
- Light sensitivity

Risk Factors for Dry Eye Syndrome

Dry eye is a chronic condition with many contributing factors, including age (it's more common for people over 40) and sex (it's more common in females). Some of the causes of dry eye, such as environment, diet and systemic disease, require a holistic approach to treatment, including dietary and environmental changes to promote a healthier ocular surface.

Environment

Our environment is a big contributor to dry eye. For example, spending a lot of time in air-conditioned or heated environments can predispose you to dry eye. Other environmental factors that promote dry eye include dust and being outside on windy days, as well as cigarette smoke — whether you are a smoker or are breathing it in secondhand.

Allergies

Allergies and dry eye are two conditions that go hand and hand. In fact, it's often difficult to tell which came first, allergies or dry eye, when a patient experiences both. Allergens such as pollen and dust can easily get trapped in the eyes and cause an allergic reaction — also known as allergic conjunctivitis. The tear film is usually able to ward off these allergens, but if you suffer from dry eye, this function is impaired and you are more likely to have an allergic reaction, such as itchy and watery eyes. Similarly, if you are suffering from allergic conjunctivitis, the inflammation present in the eye as a result of the allergic reaction releases chemicals that can disrupt the tear film and cause dry eye.

Pro Tip

Antihistamines, medications that are a common treatment for allergies, may cause dry eye as a side effect.

Medication

Many medications list dry eye as a possible side effect. Some of the most common medications that have the potential to cause or exacerbate dry eye include antihistamines, tricyclic antidepressants, diuretics, beta-blockers, hormone replacement therapy and chemotherapy.

Hormonal Changes

Menopause can increase your risk for dry eye. In fact, women over 50 have a 50% greater risk of dry eye than men of the same age. Pregnancy and oral contraceptives are also risk factors for dry eye.

Systemic Disease

Many systemic diseases are associated with a higher risk for dry eye. The most common is Sjogren's syndrome, a chronic autoimmune disease that affects the lacrimal gland (tear gland), salivary glands and other organs in the body. Other culprits include hyperthyroidism or hypothyroidism, type 1 or type 2 diabetes, rheumatoid arthritis, hormonal imbalance, lupus, rosacea, environmental allergies and psoriasis.

Eye Surgery

Having eye surgery, such as LASIK or cataract surgery, can increase your risk for dry eye or increase the severity of preexisting dry eye. If you are planning to have eye surgery, talk to your surgeon or optometrist about treating dry eye *before* the surgery. They will also advise you what to expect in terms of dry eye symptoms after surgery.

Contact Lenses

Wearing contact lenses can increase your risk for dry eye. Wearing them more than the recommended number of hours a day, as prescribed by your eye doctor, or not changing them frequently enough can make dry eye worse.

Reading and Watching TV

Our blink rate decreases from 17 times per minute to about 10 times per minute when we read or watch TV. A low blink rate gives your tears more opportunity to evaporate and can be an aggravating factor for dry eye.

Screen Time

The prevalence of dry eye increases with prolonged screen use. These days, with the abundance of smartphones, tablets and computers in our lives, we are spending more time than ever

DID YOU KNOW?

Eyelid Conditions

Blepharitis and Meibomian gland dysfunction are two common disorders of the eyelids that contribute to dry eye. These conditions are discussed in detail on page 50.

DID YOU KNOW?

Screen Time for Kids

With an increase in technology use at a younger age, we are starting to see an increase in the diagnosis of dry eye in younger people, including children. It is common to stare at our devices, and the result is that our blink rate decreases when we are using technology.

Cosmetics and Dry Eye

Sleeping in your eye makeup is a habit that can increase inflammation in your eyes and cause premature wrinkles and aging. It can also increase your risk for a sty, an infection in your eyelid, by providing an optimal breeding ground for bacteria. Another eyelid condition that can be caused or aggravated by improperly removed eye makeup is demodex, tiny mites that invade eyelashes and cause symptoms of irritated and burning eyes.

Removing your eye makeup regularly and properly can help relieve symptoms of dry eye, leave your eyes feeling fresher and help them appear whiter. Follow these simple tips for removing your eye makeup effectively:

- Choose an eye makeup remover that contains natural ingredients and is safe for ophthalmic use.
- Use an oil-based product with a cotton swab. This will allow you to remove eyeliner without scrubbing and stretching the skin around your eyelids, which can increase wrinkles.
- Avoid using baby shampoo to remove eye makeup, as it contains preservatives that can cause eye allergies, and prolonged use can lead to inflammation.

looking at screens and less time being active or resting our eyes. As a result, we're not blinking as much, and our tears are evaporating before our eyes can use them for lubrication.

Diagnosing Dry Eye Syndrome

In most cases, an optometrist or ophthalmologist can diagnose dry eye syndrome by looking at your eyes with a high-powered microscope. A detailed patient history, including a description of the symptoms and their duration, is important in the diagnosis. Another diagnostic option is the Schirmer tear test, which involves inserting a strip of special paper into your lower lid and quantifying the tears that are produced over a certain length of time.

Dry eye can also be diagnosed by an assessment of the health and integrity of the cells in the cornea. Your optometrist may instill special eye drops, such as fluorescein and lissamine green, that will show damage to the epithelial cells (the top layer) of the cornea, which is often caused by dry eye syndrome.

Dry Eye Questionnaires

Because dry eye is largely a disease characterized by symptoms, it is important for your eye doctor to have an objective way to evaluate your symptoms. As part of your evaluation, they may use a validated questionnaire, such as the Ocular Surface

Disease Index (OSDI), the McMonnies questionnaire, the Dry Eye Questionnaire 5 (DEQ-5) or the Standard Patient Evaluation of Eye Dryness (SPEED) questionnaire. These questionnaires ask you to rate the severity of a variety of ocular symptoms.

Tear Osmolarity

Osmolarity is a measure of solid particles in a solution. Most patients with dry eye have hyperosmolarity of their tear film, or a higher concentration of salt and less water in their tears than in typical tears. When measuring osmolarity, a small sample of tears is obtained. Measuring tear osmolarity is useful as an aid for diagnosing dry eye and to monitor the efficacy of treatment; however, it should not be used in isolation for a dry eye diagnosis.

Evaluation of Meibomian Glands

The Meibomian glands, which run up and down in our eyelids, produce the lipid layer of the tear film. Your optometrist or ophthalmologist can examine the consistency of the oils secreted by these glands. Ideally, the lipids have a consistency similar to that of olive oil. In cases of dry eye, the lipids often appear thicker and have a paste-like consistency.

> **Eyefood Focus**
> Curcumin, an active ingredient in the spice turmeric, has been shown to have a potential therapeutic effect in treating dry eye. Eating turmeric with black pepper increases the body's absorption of curcumin.

Current Treatments

There are many treatment options available for dry eye syndrome, depending on the cause and severity of the condition. The most important factor in the success of dry eye treatment is patient compliance. Many people find the treatment too much trouble and do not follow through with their doctor's recommendations. This can lead to frustration and discouragement for both the patient and the doctor.

If you think you may have dry eye syndrome, discuss your treatment options with your eye doctor. Be aware that treatment will be an involved process and may require frequent follow-up visits. But with patience and perseverance, the following treatments can decrease the symptoms of dry eye syndrome:

- Artificial teardrops
- Eyelid hygiene such as warm eye masks and eyelid scrubs (a special product to cleanse the eyelids)
- Anti-inflammatory medications (such as Restasis, Xiidra or mild steroid eye drops)
- Increased intake of omega-3 fatty acids (preferably from cold-water fish sources)
- Punctal occlusion (blocking tear ducts to decrease tear drainage)

Some clinics now offer comprehensive dry eye programs that include advanced treatment options:

- **Meibomian gland expression:** Used to both diagnose and treat dry eye, expression of the Meibomian glands is done in your doctor's office by applying pressure to the eyelid. Advanced systems that apply thermal pulsation to the Meibomian glands, to heat the glands and express their secretions, are also available as treatment options. Studies of one of these treatments, called Lipiflow, have shown that symptoms may be improved for up to 9 to 12 months after a single treatment. Other currently available treatments include Intense Pulse Light Treatment (IPL) and iLux.

- **Scleral contact lenses:** Although traditional contact lenses can exacerbate dry eye symptoms, a special type called scleral lenses are designed to protect the ocular surface. A well-fitted lens will provide clear vision and the comfort of a soft contact lens.

Committing to a Treatment Plan

In my optometric practice, I see patients every day who are suffering from dry eye syndrome. Some people are looking for a quick cure for their symptoms. What they do not realize is that dry eye syndrome is a chronic disease and its symptoms are a sign of inflammation in the eye. Just as it takes time for dry eye syndrome to cause discomfort, burning or watering of the eyes, so does the treatment take time to be effective.

Developing habits that will promote a healthy ocular surface is essential for achieving optimal control of dry eye. I often tell my patients, "Motivation is what gets you started; habit is what keeps you going."

A Holistic Dry Eye Treatment Plan

Every patient has unique treatment needs, but I believe a holistic approach to treating dry eye should include treatment strategies for achieving four pillars of eye health:

1. Maintain a healthy ocular surface.
2. Control your environment.
3. Improve your nutrition.
4. Make it a habit.

Maintain a Healthy Ocular Surface

- Try artificial teardrops or prescription eye drops, such as corticosteroids (to be used short-term), Restasis or Xiidra.

- Use a warm compress, such as a heated eye mask, to help improve the consistency of the lipids produced by your Meibomian glands. To be effective, warm compresses must be used consistently and must maintain a consistent heat. Your eye doctor may also recommend in-office treatments, such as Lipiflow, IPL or iLux.

- Cleanse your eyelids. Lid hygiene is recommended if patients have blepharitis (inflammation of the eyelids). There are many lid-cleansing products available. Be gentle, to avoid irritating the ocular surface.

- Increase the humidity of the ocular surface with moisture chamber goggles. When outdoors, wear sunglasses with moisture cups that fit securely around your eyes, for protection from dust and wind. Clear moisture chamber goggles are available for use inside.

Control Your Environment

- Maintain high humidity in your environment. This is an important change in treating dry eye, especially in areas with heating or air-conditioning. Use a small humidifier in your office and at home, in the rooms where you spend most of your time.

- Avoid the use of fans, including ceiling fans, as they can aggravate dry eye.

- Ensure your computer screen is below your line of sight to minimize tear evaporation.

- Take frequent screen breaks and remember to blink when reading or using a device.

- Avoid smoking cigarettes and areas where there is secondhand smoke.

Improve Your Nutrition

- Eat cold-water fish, such as salmon, rainbow trout, sardines or mackerel, three to four times per week. Omega-3 fatty acids from fish sources (DHA and EPA) are useful in the treatment of dry eye thanks to their anti-inflammatory properties.

- Reduce your intake of foods that are high in omega-6 fatty acids and promote inflammation, such as processed foods and sugary treats.

DID YOU KNOW?

Omega-3 Supplements

Supplementation with omega-3 fatty acids is often recommended for dry eye treatment. However, the optimal dosing is still being debated in the scientific literature.

- Increase your intake of GLA (gamma-linolenic acid), a beneficial omega-6 fatty acid with anti-inflammatory properties. GLA can be found in hemp seeds, oats, barley and spirulina. When eaten in combination with DHA and EPA, it has been shown to be effective in the treatment of dry eye.

Make It a Habit

Motivation is what gets you started. Habit is what keeps you going. To form a habit, psychologists say a behavior must be done consistently for 21 days. To help you follow your dry eye treatment plan, try keeping a journal to track your treatments, including eye drops, compresses, dietary changes and doctor's appointments. Your journal could include:

- A daily checklist for eye drops and ointments, warm compresses and lid care treatments
- A notation of when to take your omega-3 supplements, or a place to check off when you take them
- Recipes for eyefood smoothies (see pages 138–149)
- Articles and informative pamphlets that explain the causes of and treatments for dry eye

When eaten in combination with DHA and EPA, GLA has been shown to be effective in the treatment of dry eye.

In Summary

- Dry eye syndrome is a common chronic eye condition that affects people of all ages with varying degrees of severity.
- Dry eye syndrome does not cause vision loss, but it can cause fluctuating vision, making reading more difficult. Untreated moderate to severe dry eye can affect a person's quality of life.
- The symptoms of dry eye syndrome vary depending on its cause and severity.
- People with dry eye syndrome will often experience eye watering.
- Environmental factors can affect the severity of the symptoms.
- Omega-3 fatty acids from cold-water fish can help relieve dry eye syndrome.
- Patience is required in the treatment of dry eye syndrome, but with proper care and dietary adjustments, the symptoms can be greatly reduced.

Eyelid Disorders

Blepharitis and meibomianitis are common chronic disorders of the eyelid that are often associated with dry eye syndrome. Blepharitis is an inflammation of the eyelid margin. Meibomianitis is inflammation of the oil glands in the eyelid. Blepharitis and meibomianitis usually occur together. They are chronic conditions for which there is no cure. However, ongoing treatment can minimize the signs and symptoms of both disorders.

In people with these eyelid disorders, the oil glands in the eyelids do not function properly. As a result, the eyelids become inflamed and the normal bacteria that reside on the eyelashes proliferate. If left untreated, severe eyelid disorders can lead to the development of sties, chalazia (chronic sties) or corneal ulcers caused by sensitivity to the staphylococcal bacteria found on the eyelid.

Signs and Symptoms: Eyelid Disorders

- Eyelid redness
- Burning
- Discomfort
- Foreign body sensation (feeling like something is in your eye)
- Watery eyes
- Discharge (mucus or "sleep" in the eyes, especially in the morning)

Current Treatments

There are various courses of treatment for blepharitis and meibomianitis, depending on the severity and type of eyelid disorder. Most treatment regimens include applying warm compresses to the upper and lower eyelids for 5 to 10 minutes at least once a day, followed by eyelid hygiene using a special product to cleanse the eyelid margins. These procedures help to control the buildup of oils and bacteria at the eyelid margins. Other treatments include:

- Artificial teardrops
- Adding omega-3 fatty acids to your diet
- Anti-inflammatory eye drops or combination anti-inflammatory/antibiotic eye drops (short-term therapy)

- Oral antibiotics (used for their anti-inflammatory properties)
- In-office treatments that express and provide care for the Meibomian glands, such as Lipiflow, IPL and iLux.

Because the symptoms of eyelid disorders occur only after the inflammation, treatment takes time. It is important to continue your treatment regimen even when the symptoms have lessened and your eyes feel better. Maintaining healthy eyes takes commitment. If you currently have an eyelid disorder, the first step is making a few easy changes to your daily routine and diet.

Inflammation in the Body

The symptoms of dry eye syndrome, blepharitis and meibomianitis are the result of inflammation in the eye. Without treatment, these conditions cause inflammation on the surface of the eye. In many cases, inflammation is important to our health. It is the body's natural response to injury or foreign invaders, such as bacteria or viruses. Inflammation is the cornerstone of healing. However, in autoimmune diseases such as rheumatoid arthritis, lupus and ankylosing spondylitis, inflammation can occur for no beneficial reason.

Many factors in the North American lifestyle lead to chronic inflammation in the body. Smoking, obesity and an imbalance in our dietary intake of omega-6 and omega-3 fatty acids are all considered to be pro-inflammatory. Chronic inflammation is a risk factor in diseases such as atherosclerosis, type 2 diabetes and even cancer.

In Summary

- Blepharitis and meibomianitis are common eyelid disorders that are chronic in nature.
- There is no cure for blepharitis and meibomianitis, but daily treatment routines can minimize or eliminate their symptoms.
- Though there are many contributing factors, the underlying cause of all eyelid disorders is inflammation.
- Because omega-3 fatty acids are anti-inflammatory, they may help treat blepharitis and meibomianitis.
- Routine follow-up appointments are important in the treatment of eyelid disorders. In certain cases, oral medications may be necessary.
- Be patient. With proper treatment, the symptoms of eyelid disorders can improve greatly.

Glaucoma

Glaucoma is a disease that causes damage to the optic nerve over time. If left untreated, it may lead to loss of peripheral vision and, ultimately, tunnel vision. With regular eye exams, glaucoma can be detected at early stages. Although there is no cure for glaucoma, with ongoing treatment, vision loss can be prevented. Once vision loss occurs, it cannot be reversed, so early detection and treatment of glaucoma are critical.

According to the 2012 report "Vision Problems in the U.S.," the number of people over 40 with glaucoma increased by 22% in 10 years. The report also states that half of the people with glaucoma do not know they have the disease. To ensure early detection of glaucoma, it is important to have regular eye exams with an optometrist or ophthalmologist that include a thorough eye health assessment.

There are three types of glaucoma: primary open-angle glaucoma, normal-tension glaucoma and narrow-angle glaucoma, which can take the form of acute angle-closure glaucoma or chronic narrow-angle glaucoma.

The part of the eye where the cornea meets the iris forms an angle that functions as a drainage channel for aqueous humor (the fluid in the anterior chamber, or front part, of the eye). If the angle is normal, there is adequate space between the cornea and the iris, and enough room for the aqueous humor to drain out of the anterior chamber. If the angle is narrow, there is only a small amount of space for the aqueous humor to drain. If more aqueous humor is being produced than can be drained, intraocular pressure may increase and cause glaucoma.

Pro Tip

Once vision is lost as a result of glaucoma, it cannot be regained. However, with early detection and treatment, vision loss can be prevented.

Primary Open-Angle Glaucoma

Primary open-angle glaucoma is the most common type of glaucoma and has no symptoms in its early stages. In primary open-angle glaucoma, there is either an increased production of aqueous humor or decreased drainage of aqueous humor, despite a normal angle. Both of these circumstances can cause an increase in intraocular pressure (IOP), which can damage the optic nerve and lead to progressive loss of peripheral vision.

There are no symptoms of early primary open-angle glaucoma. As the disease progresses, blind spots may appear in the peripheral vision. However, this peripheral vision loss is not noticeable until the disease is quite advanced and the damage to the optic nerve severe. If you are at high risk of developing glaucoma, your optometrist or ophthalmologist will closely monitor your IOP, optic nerve health and peripheral vision so that they can detect and treat glaucoma before it progresses to the point where it causes vision loss.

Pro Tip

In general, normal eye pressure is between 12 and 21 mmHg (millimeters of mercury).

Risk Factors: Primary Open-Angle Glaucoma

- Family history
- Diabetes
- Migraines
- Ocular hypertension (higher-than-normal IOP)
- Age (over 40)
- History of eye injury
- Thin corneas

Diagnosing Primary Open-Angle Glaucoma

An optometrist or ophthalmologist can diagnose glaucoma during an eye examination. They will start by identifying any risk factors you may have for developing the disease, including a family history of glaucoma. During a thorough eye health exam, they will measure your intraocular pressure and examine your optic nerve for signs of damage. If you have risk factors such as higher-than-normal IOP or your optic nerve is showing possible signs of damage, they may request additional testing. These tests could include an assessment of your peripheral vision (a visual field test) and advanced imaging of your optic nerve.

Below are descriptions of the various tests used to diagnose glaucoma. A diagnosis is made only after your eye doctor reviews the results of all of the tests. Diagnosing glaucoma is not simple; your doctor must interpret the results of many tests and make clinical judgements.

DID YOU KNOW?

Case History

Collecting information about your past eye health, general health and family history is an important part of any eye health examination. Aspects of your history that could increase your risk for glaucoma include having blood relatives with glaucoma, taking steroid medications and a history of ocular trauma.

Intraocular Pressure Measurement

IOP measurement, also known as tonometry, is a part of every comprehensive eye examination. An IOP above 21 mmHg — called ocular hypertension — is a risk factor for glaucoma. If you have a high IOP measurement, your eye doctor may have you return for a follow-up to repeat the measurement.

Intraocular pressure is tolerated differently by different people. One person might tolerate an IOP of 25 with no damage to their optic nerve, while another may develop glaucoma with the same IOP. Conversely, someone with an IOP of 15 might, nevertheless, have optic nerve damage and glaucoma (see "Normal-Tension Glaucoma," page 56).

Gonioscopy

Gonioscopy is a diagnostic exam in which a lens is placed on the eye to view the angle and determine whether it is an open-angle or a narrow-angle. A narrow angle increases your risk for narrow-angle glaucoma (see page 56).

Pachymetry

Pachymetry measures the thickness of your cornea. Corneal thickness affects your IOP measurement, so this information is important for the interpretation of your IOP. Thin corneas have a lower-than-normal IOP measurement; thick corneas have a higher-than-normal measurement.

Retinal Examination

An important part of glaucoma diagnosis occurs with examination of the optic nerve during a retinal exam. Your eye doctor will look at your retina using a high-powered microscope and specialty lenses. In glaucoma, the optic nerve becomes damaged and the cup-to-disc ratio of the nerve increases. An optic nerve is like a donut with a hole in the center. The hole in the center of your optic nerve is called the cup, and the nerve itself is the disc. If the cup gets bigger over time, it may be a sign of glaucoma.

Visual Field Testing (Perimetry)

Visual field testing is a detailed test that determines whether you have any loss or decrease in your peripheral vision. To perform this test, you will have a patch over one eye and look at a target straight ahead. Without moving your eye from the central target, you will be asked to click a button every time you see a light in your peripheral vision. Because this test measures the sensitivity of your peripheral vision, some lights will be dim and others will be bright. The test randomly shines lights in various locations, at different intensities, to determine the dimmest light you can see in each area. During the test, it is important to maintain your gaze straight ahead at the target; if you move your eye, the test will not be reliable.

Because it is an objective test, many people find visual field testing difficult, as they feel like they want to move their eye from the central gaze, or that they are missing lights. It may help to know that, to be accurate, visual field tests should be repeatable. That means, if you have a loss of visual field (a visual field defect), it will appear in two tests done at different times. So don't be surprised if your eye doctor has you repeat a visual field test on another day. Once glaucoma is diagnosed, visual field testing is usually repeated every 4 to 6 months to monitor for any changes in peripheral vision.

Imaging Technology

The purpose of imaging technology in glaucoma is to monitor the loss of optic nerve fibers. In glaucoma, the nerve fiber layer gets thinner over time. Advanced imaging measures the thickness of the nerve fiber layer; if it is thinning over time, this can be a sign that glaucoma is developing or progressing. There are different types of optic nerve imaging available, including optical coherence tomography (OCT), Heidelberg retinal tomography (HRT) and the GDx Nerve Fiber Analyzer.

Current Treatments for Primary Open-Angle Glaucoma

In most cases, glaucoma is a disease that progresses slowly, so your eye doctor may choose to monitor your eyes closely for some time before starting treatment. Treatments currently available include prescription eye drops, laser surgery and traditional surgery.

Eye Drops

Prescription eye drops are the most common treatment for early glaucoma. Eye drops reduce IOP by either increasing the flow of aqueous humor out of the anterior chamber or decreasing the production of aqueous humor. Different eye drops have different dosing schedules, from once daily to three or four times per day. Early glaucoma is often managed by taking one drop, once a day. If intraocular pressure is not controlled with a single eye drop, multiple eye drops can be taken together.

Tell your eye doctor if your prescription eye drops bother your eyes. You may have an allergy to that particular medication. There are many medications available to treat glaucoma, so if you develop side effects (such as red, itchy or burning eyes) while taking eye drops, your doctor can prescribe another type that you might tolerate better.

> ### • CAUTION •
>
> Certain medications can interact with some glaucoma medications. It is important to tell your eye doctor about *all* the medications you take.

How to Insert Eye Drops

1. Tilt your head back.
2. Pull down your lower eyelid.
3. Tip the bottle upside down and instill the drop into the area within your lower lid.
4. Repeat steps 2 and 3 with your other eye.
5. Close your eyes and use your fingertips to put light pressure on your tear ducts (in your inner eyelids, near your nose) for 2 minutes. This is called punctual occlusion and will keep the eye drops in your eyes and prevent them from being absorbed into your body.

Laser Surgery

Selective laser trabeculoplasty (SLT) can be used to lower IOP in primary open-angle glaucoma or secondary open-angle glaucoma (see FAQ, page 58). It can be used as an initial treatment, instead of eye drops, or as an additional treatment when eye drops are not controlling IOP sufficiently.

Surgery

Trabeculectomy surgery lowers IOP in patients by making a filter, or bleb, in the sclera, allowing the aqueous humor to drain through. This surgery is usually performed only if medications and laser surgery can no longer control IOP. It will lower IOP but will not restore any vision that has already been lost.

Normal-Tension Glaucoma

In some circumstances, damage to the optic nerve and loss of peripheral vision occur when the IOP is normal. This is called normal-tension glaucoma or low-pressure glaucoma. The Beaver Dam Eye Study, a study funded by the National Eye Institute to collect information on the prevalence and incidence of common eye diseases, reported that nearly one-third of cases of glaucoma are normal-tension. Researchers aren't certain of the exact cause of optic nerve damage when the IOP is normal. A current theory posits that blood flow to the optic nerve is compromised, causing damage to the nerve and subsequent loss of peripheral vision.

Normal-tension glaucoma has also been associated with migraine headaches, Raynaud's disease (a condition where there is reduced blood flow to smaller arteries, such as those in the hands and feet) and autoimmune diseases.

As for open-angle glaucoma, eye drops are the first line of treatment for normal-tension glaucoma.

> Normal-tension glaucoma is more prevalent in Japan and Korea. It affects women more often than men.

Narrow-Angle Glaucoma

There are two types of narrow-angle glaucoma: acute angle-closure glaucoma and chronic narrow-angle glaucoma. Acute angle closure is an ocular emergency and may present with severe ocular symptoms such as blurred vision, eye pain or headaches. Chronic narrow-angle glaucoma occurs when the angle is narrowed but not completely closed. Unlike acute angle-closure glaucoma, chronic narrow-angle glaucoma usually has no symptoms.

Acute Angle-Closure Glaucoma

Acute angle-closure glaucoma occurs when the drainage channel of the eye becomes blocked, causing a spike in eye pressure. An IOP spike can damage the optic nerve and result in peripheral vision loss, but early treatment can prevent both nerve damage and vision loss.

Unlike open-angle glaucoma, which is asymptomatic, acute angle-closure glaucoma has symptoms that include ocular pain and loss of vision. If you experience symptoms of acute angle-closure glaucoma, contact your eye doctor right away.

Signs and Symptoms: Acute Angle-Closure Glaucoma

- Sudden blurry vision
- Severe eye pain
- Headache
- Nausea
- Vomiting
- Seeing halos around lights

Chronic Narrow-Angle Glaucoma

Unlike the acute form of narrow-angle glaucoma, chronic narrow-angle glaucoma can cause slow progression of vision loss over time without symptoms. Your optometrist or ophthalmologist will diagnose narrow-angle glaucoma by examining your anterior chamber (the front part of your eye) and measuring your IOP. They may also perform gonioscopy (see page 54) to view the angle of your eye in detail.

Risk Factors: Narrow-Angle Glaucoma

- **Age:** As we age, the lens in our eyes gets larger and the drainage channels may get smaller, increasing the risk for both acute angle-closure and chronic narrow-angle glaucoma. Removing the lens through cataract surgery can decrease the risk.
- **Race:** Asian and Inuit people have an increased risk.
- **Sex:** Women have a higher risk than men.
- **Farsightedness:** People who are farsighted are more likely to have narrow angles, which can increase their risk for an acute angle-closure attack or chronic narrow-angle glaucoma. Farsighted eyes tend to be smaller than average, and angle closure is more common in smaller eyes.
- **Family history:** Having blood relatives with the disease increases your risk of developing it.

Current Treatments

Treatments for narrow-angle glaucoma include:

- **Eye drops or oral medications:** The initial treatment usually involves lowering IOP through the use of eye drops or pills. This treatment will often be done in-office, and your IOP will be monitored until it decreases to a normal level.

- **Laser surgery:** Peripheral iridotomy makes a small hole in your iris to create another avenue for the aqueous humor to drain out of the anterior chamber. It is often performed to prevent angle-closure glaucoma in people who have anatomically narrow angles.

- **Surgery:** In some cases, filtration surgery or removal of the lens (cataract surgery) may be required to treat narrow-angle glaucoma.

FAQ

Q. What is secondary glaucoma?

A. Secondary glaucoma can be open-angle or narrow-angle glaucoma, and refers to any type of glaucoma with a known cause, such as trauma, inflammation, steroid use, advanced cataracts or diabetes. Other types of secondary glaucoma include pseudoexfoliative glaucoma (where IOP becomes elevated by a protein-like substance that is produced in high amounts in the eye), pigmentary dispersion glaucoma (when pigment sloughs off the back of the iris and clogs the drainage channel), neovascular glaucoma (caused by new blood vessel growth over the iris and in the angle; can occur in uncontrolled diabetic retinopathy and other retinal conditions), uveitic glaucoma (caused by inflammatory conditions of the eye) and congenital glaucoma (a rare condition caused by abnormal development of the drainage channels of the eye).

Nutrition and Glaucoma

Lowering IOP with eye drops, laser surgery or traditional surgery is the standard care for treating glaucoma; however, patients and doctors have shown an interest in whether nutrition and lifestyle factors can help with the management of the disease. Although more research is needed in this area, early scientific studies have shown a possible protective effect from certain foods and drinks:

- **Fruits and vegetables:** Some studies have shown a decreased likelihood of developing glaucoma in women who consumed a diet high in fruits and vegetables that contain vitamin A, vitamin C and carotenes. In addition, eating leafy green vegetables has been shown to be protective against glaucoma.

- **Tea:** Early research shows that people who drink tea may have less risk of developing glaucoma. Tea is high in polyphenols and flavonoids, which may help reduce oxidative stress and improve blood flow.
- **Ginkgo biloba:** Studies have demonstrated that ginkgo biloba, a tree native to China, can increase ocular blood flow, increase retinal ganglion cell survival and reduce oxidative stress. As normal-tension glaucoma is thought to be caused by a reduction in ocular blood flow, ginkgo biloba may prove to be protective, although further investigation is needed.

Nutrition Advice for People with or at Risk for Glaucoma

These nutrition tips may complement a treatment plan from your eye doctor; however, nutritional management of glaucoma does not replace medical management. Be sure to ask your eye doctor about the relationship between nutrition and glaucoma.

- Maintain a healthy weight.
- Eat a diet high in vegetables and fruit.
- Consume leafy green vegetables, such as spinach, kale, collard greens and dandelion greens, daily.
- Enjoy a daily cup of tea.

A New Glaucoma Theory

The long-standing theory about the cause of glaucoma is that elevated intraocular pressure causes mechanical damage to the optic nerve. But newer scientific research suggests that ocular perfusion pressure (OPP) — mean blood pressure minus intraocular pressure — may play a role. This vascular theory suggests that if OPP gets too low, blood flow to the optic nerve is compromised. Researchers believe that OPP may change drastically throughout the day, and that these variations, if severe, may cause damage in some people. Certain people will be more susceptible to low OPP.

Medical Cannabis

According to the American Academy of Ophthalmology, marijuana ingested by pill or inhaled by smoking has been shown to lower IOP; however, the effect lasts only 3 to 4 hours. These effects were first reported in 1971. Typical glaucoma medications last 12 to 24 hours. To be effective, marijuana would need to be taken every 3 to 4 hours, which would cause cognitive impairment and leave a person unable to drive.

In addition, scientists believe that damage to the optic nerve from glaucoma is caused by reduced blood flow to the optic nerve. Marijuana decreases blood pressure throughout the body, so any potential benefit from reduced eye pressure would be canceled out by decreased blood flow to the optic nerve.

Smoking anything is generally bad for eye health, increasing the risk for AMD and causing dry eye, and topical marijuana preparations have not been effective and cause irritation.

In Summary

- Glaucoma is a disease that causes loss of peripheral vision over time.
- Primary open-angle glaucoma, normal-tension glaucoma and chronic narrow-angle glaucoma do not cause any symptoms.
- Acute angle-closure glaucoma is an ocular emergency that requires immediate treatment to lower the intraocular pressure. Symptoms of acute angle-closure glaucoma include blurry vision, eye pain and headache.
- Treatments for glaucoma include eye drops, laser surgery and traditional surgery.

FAQ

Q. Do high blood pressure and cardiovascular disease have any effect on my eyes?

A. High blood pressure, high cholesterol and diabetes can affect the health of your eyes by causing damage to the retina. The blood vessels in the retina are some of the smallest in the body; as a result, the eye is one of the first organs to be affected by chronic high blood pressure or diabetes. It is important to have your eyes checked yearly if you have cardiovascular disease or diabetes. Your optometrist will do a dilated retinal exam and digital imaging of your retina to detect early signs of changes. Early detection of retinopathy may prevent future vision loss.

Current scientific research also shows that cardiovascular disease and AMD share many of the same risk factors, including age, smoking, antioxidant levels, physical activity, body mass index and waist circumference. Because of this connection, many similarities exist between a heart-friendly and an eye-friendly lifestyle. Good nutrition, physical activity, maintaining a healthy weight and not smoking will promote both healthy eyes and a healthy heart.

Most people can paint a picture of a heart-friendly lifestyle. The next piece of the puzzle is to reinforce that a healthy heart, healthy eyes and a healthy body are all connected.

Diabetes and Eye Health

Diabetes is the leading cause of new cases of blindness among adults aged 20 to 74. The National Eye Institute reports that nearly half of Americans with diabetes have diabetic retinopathy. Of those, nearly 5% have sight-threatening retinopathy. According to the Canadian National Institute for the Blind, diabetes is the leading cause of blindness in Canadians under 50. There are 500,000 Canadians affected by diabetic retinopathy, and the risk of blindness in people with diabetes is up to 25 times more than for people without diabetes.

Data from the 2011 "National Diabetes Fact Sheet" show that nearly 26 million Americans have been diagnosed with diabetes. Another 79 million are considered prediabetic and are at risk for developing the disease. In addition, 7 million Americans suffer from the disease but remain undiagnosed. According to Diabetes Canada, 11 million Canadians are living with diabetes or prediabetes.

Type 2 diabetes is preventable, and it accounts for up to 95% of all cases of diabetes.

- **Prediabetes** is diagnosed when your blood sugar is higher than normal, but not high enough to warrant a diagnosis of diabetes. Prediabetes can develop into type 2 diabetes; however, with lifestyle and nutrition changes, it can also be reversed. It can occur at any age.

- **Type 1 diabetes** includes 5% of all cases of diabetes. It is a condition in which the pancreas does not produce insulin. Type 1 diabetes can be diagnosed at any age.

- **Type 2 diabetes** is the most common form of diabetes and accounts for 90% to 95% of all cases. It occurs when the body develops insulin resistance and cannot use insulin properly. Initially, the body can produce more insulin to make up for this dysfunction; however, eventually it is unable to keep up, and type 2 diabetes develops.

One of the most alarming aspects of these statistics is the increasing frequency of both type 1 and type 2 diabetes in North American youth. Between 2009 and 2011, the incidence of both conditions increased by more than 20%.

This is a real health crisis. However, the good news is that we can do something about it. Type 2 diabetes is preventable, and it accounts for up to 95% of all cases of diabetes. If we educate ourselves about the relationship between weight, exercise, dietary intake and diabetic eye disease, and take action to make better everyday health choices, we can reduce the incidence of type 2 diabetes and help prevent associated vision loss.

DID YOU KNOW?

Blurry Vision

A common symptom of chronic elevated blood glucose is blurry vision. This occurs when there is a change in your refractive error (corrective lens prescription) so that your sight is blurry with your usual correction. This change is temporary and will revert when your blood glucose levels are controlled.

Risk Factors for Type 2 Diabetes

Excess weight gain is one of the fundamental causes of type 2 diabetes. Indeed, the risk of developing diabetes increases sevenfold in overweight people and twenty- to forty-fold in obese people. The most widely accepted way to determine a patient's weight status is to calculate body mass index (BMI), which is a ratio based on weight and height.

Waist circumference is another predictor of diabetes. According to a cohort of the Nurses' Health Study, the risk of type 2 diabetes increased progressively in patients with the largest waist circumferences — 35 inches (87.5 cm) or greater in women; 40 inches (100 cm) or greater in men.

According to the Harvard T.H. Chan School of Public Health, losing 7% to 10% of your current weight can reduce your chances of developing type 2 diabetes by as much as 50%. For example, someone who weighs 150 pounds (68 kg) would need to lose just 10 to 15 pounds (4.5 to 6.8 kg). For patients who don't exercise or who have poor diets, this weight reduction goal is relatively easy to achieve with some straightforward lifestyle changes.

Losing 7% to 10% of your current weight can reduce your chances of developing type 2 diabetes by as much as 50%.

Signs and Symptoms: Type 2 Diabetes

Symptoms of high blood glucose and undiagnosed diabetes include:

- Excess thirst, hunger and urination
- Weight loss
- Infections
- Slow wound healing
- Fatigue
- Blurry vision

Current Treatments for Type 1 and Type 2 Diabetes

The three main pillars of diabetes treatment are medication, exercise and nutrition.

Medication

Type 1 diabetes is treated with insulin injections through syringes, pens or an insulin pump. Blood glucose levels must be monitored regularly to ensure that the insulin is being properly administered. It is important to work closely with your doctors and health care team to determine the best type of insulin and dosage for you.

Type 2 diabetes is treated with oral medications and sometimes insulin to control blood glucose levels.

Exercise

Regular exercise will help you maintain more stable blood glucose levels and a healthy weight. Talk to your doctor before starting any new exercise regimen. Your blood glucose may drop during physical activity, so ask your health care team about the best times to exercise.

Regular exercise will help you maintain more stable blood glucose levels and a healthy weight.

Nutrition

Food is an important part of diabetes management, because the food we ingest directly affects blood glucose levels. There is no single diet that is recommended for people with diabetes, but it is important to visit a dietitian, who will help you formulate meal plans and teach you how certain foods affect your blood glucose level.

Ocular Effects of Diabetes

If you have diabetes, have your eyes checked annually by an optometrist or ophthalmologist. Diabetes can affect your eyes in a variety of ways. Changes in your blood glucose levels can cause temporary changes in your refractive error (corrective lens prescription). Diabetic retinopathy is perhaps the best known and most serious complication of diabetes. Cataracts and dry eye syndrome are also more common in people with diabetes.

Changes in Refractive Error

Fluctuations in your blood glucose level can cause a chemical change in the composition of your lens, leading to a change in your refractive error. In fact, one of the initial symptoms of diabetes, before people are even aware they have the disease, is blurry vision. Once your blood glucose levels are controlled and return to normal, your refractive error will stabilize.

Pro Tip

If you have diabetes and your blood glucose levels have been fluctuating, it is a good idea to wait until they stabilize before you get new glasses.

Diabetic Retinopathy

The blood vessels in the retina are some of the smallest in the body; thus, they are susceptible to damage from diabetes, especially from fluctuations in blood glucose levels over time. In diabetic retinopathy, the blood vessels in the retina can leak or become blocked. In proliferative diabetic retinopathy, new blood vessels can grow in the retina.

Diabetic retinopathy can lead to vision loss. Early detection is essential, as timely treatment can reduce the risk of vision loss.

- **Non-proliferative diabetic retinopathy** is an early stage of diabetic retinopathy. It can occur at any time and is characterized by hemorrhages or deposits in the retina. Patients with non-proliferative diabetic retinopathy are encouraged to maintain better control of their blood glucose levels and to see their eye doctor every 3 to 6 months for dilated eye examinations and retinal imaging.

- **Proliferative diabetic retinopathy** incurs the greatest risk of vision loss. It may involve new blood vessel growth in the retina and large retinal or vitreous hemorrhages. In severe cases, it can lead to retinal detachment. Treatment options include laser photocoagulation of the retina, to prevent further growth of new blood vessels, or vitrectomy surgery if there is evidence of a vitreous hemorrhage or traction of the vitreous on the retina.

FAQ

Q. How can I help prevent vision loss from diabetic eye disease?

A. The best way to prevent vision loss is to visit an optometrist or ophthalmologist for a comprehensive eye examination at least once a year. Ensure that your exam includes retinal imaging, such as digital retinal photography or ocular coherence tomography (OCT). Here are some other steps you can take:

- Maintain steady and healthy blood glucose levels. See your diabetes team regularly to make sure your levels are controlled. Ensure that your doctors and other health care professionals are communicating with each other.
- Maintain healthy blood pressure and blood cholesterol levels.
- Stay physically active. For optimal health benefits, adults should exert themselves for at least 30 minutes per day. Children should engage in at least 60 continuous minutes of physical activity every day.
- Quit smoking.
- Maintain a healthy weight and follow a nutritious diet. Avoid processed foods and sugars. Eat foods high in lutein, zeaxanthin, vitamin C, vitamin E and zinc for optimal eye health.

Clinically Significant Macular Edema

Clinically significant macular edema occurs when fluid leaks into the macula (the central part of the retina). This is the most common cause of vision loss in diabetes. Symptoms include blurriness or waviness in the central vision. Clinically significant macular edema can occur on its own or with non-proliferative or proliferative diabetic retinopathy. Treatment options include laser photocoagulation and injections into the eye of corticosteroids or medications that block the protein VEGF, which is responsible for new blood vessel growth.

Nutrition Tips for People with Diabetes

The typical North American diet contains high amounts of processed, calorie-dense foods that offer little nutritional value and promote weight gain. Serving sizes, both in restaurants and at home, are expanding in direct proportion to the waistlines of millions of North Americans. Furthermore, many people, particularly children, are consuming too many soft drinks and other sugary beverages that can promote type 2 diabetes. If these general trends continue, more people will experience the signs and symptoms of diabetic eye disease at increasingly younger ages.

If you have diabetes, it is important to meet with a dietitian to create meal plans that will help you manage your blood glucose levels and maintain a healthy weight.

Follow a Meal Plan

In order to lose weight, we need to expend more calories than we consume. If you have diabetes, it is important to meet with a dietitian to create meal plans that will help you manage your blood glucose levels and maintain a healthy weight.

In general, healthy diets that promote stable blood glucose levels are rich in vegetables and fruits, and low in saturated and trans fats, sodium and added sugar. It is also important to eat three meals a day, at regular times, and to have healthy snacks at regular intervals.

Go for Whole Grains

Processed foods and refined grains make up a large portion of the average North American's diet. These foods increase blood glucose levels significantly more than healthier, non-processed alternatives.

Whole grains contain more fiber and generally have a lower glycemic index than refined grains. A diet rich in whole grains is associated with a reduced risk of type 2 diabetes, whereas a high intake of processed foods is directly linked with an increased risk of diabetic disease. Everyone should make an effort to eat whole grains in place of refined grains.

Pro Tip

Whole grains have many health benefits, but they often have just as many calories as refined grains, so be mindful of proper serving sizes.

Avoid Sugary Drinks

There is no cordial way to address this point: North Americans must stop drinking calorie-laden soft drinks! Soda, sweet tea, blended juice drinks and specialty coffees all contain large amounts of empty calories in the form of simple sugars. They have a high glycemic load and do not help us feel full so we don't consume less food at our next meal.

Multiple studies have shown that women who drank at least one sugar-sweetened soft drink or fruit punch beverage per day were at an increased risk for developing type 2 diabetes.

Eyefoods Tips: For People with Diabetes

- Fill your plate with eye-healthy fruits and vegetables, including:
  - A handful of raw leafy greens each day;
  - ½ cup (125 mL) cooked leafy greens, twice per week;
  - ½ cup (125 mL) orange vegetables (squash, carrots, pumpkin or sweet potatoes) most days;
  - 2 orange bell peppers per week (raw and cooked);
  - ½ cup (125 mL) green vegetables, such as raw and/or cooked broccoli, Brussels sprouts, green peas, green beans, asparagus and zucchini, every day;
  - Up to three servings of kiwifruit, avocado, cantaloupe, citrus fruit or berries per day. A serving is 1 medium fruit or ½ cup (125 mL).
- Avoid fruit juice and dried fruits, as they are high in sugar.
- Include whole grains in your diet daily. Good choices include quinoa, barley, whole-grain bread and whole-grain pasta. Monitor serving sizes. One serving is ½ cup (125 mL) cooked grain or pasta or 1 slice of bread.
- Choose lean meat and poultry, such as turkey breast, chicken breast and lean cuts of beef.
- Use healthy oils, such as olive oil.

In Summary

- Type 1 diabetes encompasses 5% of all diabetes.
- Type 2 diabetes accounts for 95% of all diabetes. Type 2 diabetes is preventable.
- Diabetic retinopathy is a leading cause of vision loss in adults under the age of 50 in both the United States and Canada.
- People with diabetes should have their eyes examined by an optometrist or an ophthalmologist at least once a year.
- Clinically significant macular edema is the leading cause of vision loss in people with diabetes. It occurs when fluid leaks into the macula. Treatment options include laser photocoagulation and injections of anti-VEGF medication or corticosteroids.
- Proper nutrition, maintaining a healthy weight and regular exercise are important lifestyle factors in managing diabetes.

PART 2

The Eyefoods Plan

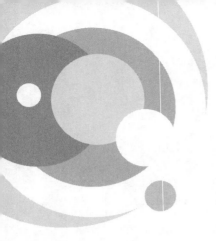

Chapter 4

Eye Nutrients

What I call "eye nutrients" are a group of nutrients that are beneficial to eye health. Nutrition is a cornerstone of eye health because certain nutrients are found in ocular tissue, and the eye uses these nutrients to function. For example, vitamin C is found in every ocular tissue, and the carotenoids lutein and zeaxanthin are found in high concentrations in the lens and retina. In fact, lutein deposits can be found 1,000 times more in the macula than anywhere else in the body.

In this chapter, I will describe the most important eye nutrients, as well as dietary factors such as glycemic index and fiber intake. We will explore the difference between macronutrients (protein, carbohydrates and fats) and micronutrients and learn why both types of nutrients are important for ocular health.

Although nutrients on their own may help to prevent eye disease, it is the synergy of nutrients that best maintains eye health. Chapters 5 and 7 will show you how to benefit from nutrient synergy through a diet high in eyefoods.

> The eye is one of the most highly metabolic organs in the body, and proper nutrition is important in ocular function and the prevention of ocular disease.

Macronutrients and General Health

The macronutrients — carbohydrates, protein and fat — are nutrients that the human body requires in large amounts on a daily basis. Some foods provide all three of the macronutrients, while others provide just one or two. Some fad diets try to restrict certain macronutrients, such as carbs or fat, while others bump up consumption of a nutrient; however, for optimal health, it is important to eat all three macronutrients in their appropriate balance every day.

Pro Tip

When choosing carbohydrates, look for foods that are high in fiber and low in sugar. Fruits, vegetables and legumes, such as beans, peas and lentils, are good choices.

Carbohydrates

Carbohydrates are found primarily in plant foods. There are three main types of carbohydrate: sugar and sugar alcohols, starches and dietary fiber. The "Dietary Guidelines for Americans" and Health Canada recommend that 45% to 65% of daily calories come from carbohydrates. That's about 225 to 235 grams per day for a 2,000-calorie diet.

FAQ

Q. How much of each nutrient do I need?

A. The recommended dosage of each nutrient varies for people with different medical conditions and for healthy individuals. For disease prevention or management, your health care professional will follow the guidelines of current scientific research to determine the appropriate amount of each nutrient for you. For healthy individuals, the Institute of Medicine (a department of the National Institutes of Health in the United States) has issued reference values for nutrient intakes, called dietary reference intakes (DRIs). Health Canada also uses DRIs to determine adequate nutrient intakes for healthy population groups that are not at high risk for disease.

Scientific studies are sometimes published that recommend nutrient doses higher than the DRIs. These often conflicting reports can cause confusion, so it is always important to discuss nutrient dosages with your health care provider.

The DRIs are made up of four values:

- **RDA (recommended dietary allowance):** The average daily intake of a nutrient that is enough to meet the dietary requirements for healthy individuals. The RDA varies according to age group and sex.

- **AI (adequate intake):** The estimated average intake of a nutrient for a healthy population. It is applicable when an RDA cannot be determined.

- **UL (tolerable upper limit):** The highest daily intake of a nutrient that is likely to have no adverse effects. The UL is dependent on sex and age group.

- **DV (daily value):** Used in nutrition facts tables, this value is set by the United States Department of Agriculture (USDA) and Health Canada to help consumers determine how much of a specific nutrient is in a food compared to their recommended intake of that nutrient. The DV can be similar to but is not always the same as the RDA of a nutrient. On a food label, the %DV indicates what percentage of the recommended DV you receive when you consume one serving of that food.

In this chapter, I will refer to the RDA, AI and UL values for eye nutrients.

The USDA and the U.S. Department of Health and Human Services (HHS) publish the "Dietary Guidelines for Americans" and Health Canada publishes "Eating Well with Canada's Food Guide" as guides to healthy daily food choices. Both guides can be found online.

Sugar and Sugar Alcohols

Sugars are found naturally in dairy, fruit and vegetables, but are also added to many of the processed foods that make up a large proportion of the North American diet.

The "Dietary Guidelines for Americans" recommends consuming less than 10% of calories per day from added sugars. According to the U.S. Food and Drug Administration (FDA), most Americans exceed the amount of recommended sugars, consuming 270 calories — or 13% of calories — from added sugars, mostly from beverages, desserts and sweets.

Health Canada recommends limiting consumption of foods that contain more than 15% of the daily value for sugar, as indicated on a food's nutrition label. Examples of foods that contain more than 15% DV of sugar are soft drinks, chocolate milk, flavored yogurt and fruit juice. Examples of foods that contain less than 15% DV of sugar include plain yogurt, white milk and unsweetened frozen fruit.

Starches

A starch is defined as many glucose molecules bound together. Examples of starches are beans, peas, grains and vegetables. Your body breaks down starches into glucose, which is used by cells to create energy.

Dietary Fiber

Like starches, dietary fiber is made up of sugar molecules linked together; the difference is that the body cannot easily digest fiber, whereas starch is easily broken down into individual glucose molecules. There are two types of dietary fiber: soluble fiber and insoluble fiber. Both types increase your satiety after a meal — they make you feel full for longer. Both the American and the Canadian guidelines suggest an intake of 25 grams of fiber per day, based on a 2,000-calorie diet.

Glycemic Index and Glycemic Load

The glycemic index (GI) is a measure of how much an individual food raises the blood glucose level as compared to a standard food (glucose or white bread). Researchers developed the concept of the glycemic index for use in the management of diabetes, where the body's glucose tolerance is disrupted. However, recent studies show that the glycemic index of foods also plays a role in other diseases, such as cardiovascular disease, cancer and age-related macular degeneration (AMD).

Foods with a high glycemic index include white bread, foods high in sugar (such as baked goods) and certain breakfast cereals. Foods with a low glycemic index include whole grains (such as barley), legumes (such as lentils) and sweet potatoes.

- **Glycemic index and eye health:** A diet rich in high-GI foods can increase the risk of cataracts and AMD. A low-GI diet promotes eye health.
- **Glycemic index and general health:** A diet rich in high-GI foods can increase the risk of type 2 diabetes, cardiovascular disease and certain types of cancer.

Glycemic load is a measure of the glycemic index of a particular food in relation to its carbohydrate content. Proponents of the glycemic load theory suggest that small portions of high-GI foods have a similar effect on glucose levels in the bloodstream as larger portions of low-GI foods.

Soluble fiber dissolves in water to form a gel-like material. It is found in beans, peas, fruits, oats, nuts, seeds and vegetables. One benefit of consuming foods high in soluble fiber is that it slows digestion, helping to prevent the rapid rise of blood glucose. It can also interfere with the absorption of dietary fat and cholesterol, and lower low-density lipoprotein (LDL) cholesterol — the "bad" cholesterol.

Insoluble fiber does not dissolve in water and passes through the digestive system intact, adding bulk to stool and speeding up the movement of food and waste through the digestive system. Eating foods high in insoluble fiber is a great way to stay "regular." Foods high in insoluble fiber include fruits, nuts, seeds, vegetables, wheat bran and whole grains such as barley, buckwheat, bulgur, millet, quinoa and brown rice.

> Food manufacturers can voluntarily list the amount in grams of soluble and insoluble fiber on food labels.

Protein

Protein is part of every cell in our body. In addition to providing energy for the body, protein is necessary for proper growth and development, and for most physiological processes, such as immune response and vision. It helps with cellular repair and is important for healing after surgery and when weight training.

Proteins are made up of amino acids. There are 20 different types of amino acids. Nine of the amino acids are considered essential, because they are not made by the body — we must get them from our diet. The remaining 11 are nonessential, as the body makes them.

Complete proteins contain all of the essential amino acids and are found in animal foods. Incomplete proteins, which do not have all of the essential amino acids, include most plant foods. Complementary proteins are two or more incomplete protein sources that, when eaten in combination at the same meal or in the same day, compensate for a lack of complete proteins. It is important for people who follow a plant-based diet to include complementary proteins in their meals. For example, you might combine beans and brown rice, or add chickpeas and nuts to a salad.

The USDA has set the daily value for protein at 50 grams per day, based on a 2,000-calorie diet. There is no daily value for protein under Canadian guidelines. Most Americans easily reach the recommended daily value, but their main protein source is meat, which tends to be higher in saturated fat.

> **Eyefood Focus**
> Lentils are a great plant-based high-protein food, with 1 cup (250 mL) of cooked lentils containing 18 grams of protein and no saturated fat. Combine lentils with sunflower or pumpkin seeds as complementary proteins.

Fat

From a health standpoint, fat often gets a bad rap. However, fat plays an important role in our bodily processes. It is part of the cell membrane and is needed for proper growth and development.

In addition to aiding in absorption of the fat-soluble vitamins A, D, E and K, it is used in blood clotting, nervous system function, reproduction and immune response. From a cuisine standpoint, fat adds taste and texture to food and makes us feel full and satisfied. However, this comes at a caloric price, as fat has more than twice as many calories per gram as carbs and protein.

The FDA and Health Canada recommend that adults consume 65 grams of fat per day, based on a 2,000-calorie diet, or 20% to 35% of calories from fat.

There are three different types of fat: unsaturated fat, saturated fat and trans fat. Most foods include a combination of both saturated and unsaturated fats, but they are characterized by the fatty acid that predominates. So, for example, olive oil is known as an unsaturated fat because it contains more unsaturated fat than saturated fat, whereas butter is called a saturated fat because it has more saturated fat than unsaturated fat.

Unsaturated Fat

Unsaturated fat is found in higher amounts in plants and is usually liquid at room temperature. There are two types of unsaturated fat: polyunsaturated fats, which are found in walnuts, flax seeds and fish; and monounsaturated fats, found in avocados, almonds, pumpkin seeds, sunflower seeds, olives and olive oil.

Both mono- and polyunsaturated fats contribute good amounts of vitamin E to our diet. They have been shown to reduce the risk of cardiovascular disease when eaten in place of saturated fat. However, all fats are a concentrated source of calories, so eat unsaturated fats in place of saturated fat rather than adding them to your diet.

Although it is not mandatory for food manufacturers to do so, poly- and monounsaturated fats are often listed on food labels.

Saturated Fat

Saturated fat is found in higher amounts in animal products, except seafood and fish, which are high in unsaturated fat. Saturated fat is usually solid at room temperature. Sources of saturated fat include beef, chicken, pork, cream, whole milk, butter and ice cream. It can raise LDL cholesterol in the blood, which can increase the risk for cardiovascular disease.

The human body makes more saturated fat than it needs, so it is not necessary for us to get it from food. In fact, most people exceed the recommended amount of saturated fat. The "Dietary Guidelines for Americans" and Health Canada recommend consuming less than 10% calories per day from saturated fat, or 20 grams for a 2,000-calorie diet.

Trans Fat

Trans fat is an unsaturated fat found primarily in hydrogenated oils. Its structure is different from unsaturated fats that are found naturally in food. Trans fat has detrimental health effects, even when consumed in small amounts. It raises LDL cholesterol and lowers HDL cholesterol (high-density lipoprotein, the "good" cholesterol), it is pro-inflammatory, and it can contribute to insulin resistance.

Historically, trans fats were used in processed foods to improve texture, shelf life and flavor stability. However, efforts have been made to reduce the amount of trans fat consumed by North Americans. As of 2006, manufacturers are required to list all trans fats on food labels, and in 2015, the FDA passed a law that bans food manufacturers from adding partially hydrogenated oils to processed foods. In Canada, trans fats are banned in all foods that are sold, including imported products and foods prepared and served in restaurants.

Micronutrients and General Health

The body requires micronutrients — vitamins and minerals — in smaller amounts than macronutrients. Micronutrients enable the body to produce enzymes, hormones and other substances responsible for proper growth and development. Although we need only small amounts, the health consequences can be severe if we are deficient in micronutrients.

Vitamins that are important for overall health include B vitamins (which aid in cell function), vitamin D (which helps the body absorb calcium) and vitamins A, C and E (which act as antioxidants). Minerals that are important for health include calcium (bone health), magnesium (normal nerve and muscle function, immune function) and zinc (cell division, wound healing and immune function).

DID YOU KNOW?

Cholesterol

Cholesterol is a waxy, fat-like substance produced mostly by the liver. It is found in all cells of the body. Dietary cholesterol is found only in animal products, including beef, chicken and pork fat, cream and milk, butter, egg yolks and shellfish. In both the United States and Canada, the daily value for cholesterol is less than 300 milligrams per day.

DID YOU KNOW?

Vitamin C Deficiency

The disease scurvy is caused by a diet lacking in vitamin C. This fact was known as early as the 15th century, when sailors would often lose their lives due to scurvy, which they developed because fresh produce was unavailable while they were at sea for long periods of time.

FAQ

Q. What are phytonutrients?

A. Phytonutrients are chemical compounds found in plant foods. Although they are not necessary for human life, they may help prevent disease and assist with bodily functions. There are 25,000 phytonutrients in nature. Examples of phytonutrients that may be beneficial to overall health are carotenoids (including lutein, zeaxanthin, beta-carotene and lycopene), flavonoids (found in dark chocolate) and resveratrol (found in red wine and skin of red grapes).

Top Nutrients for Eye Health

Research shows that nutrition may have an impact on some ocular diseases, such as age-related macular degeneration (AMD), cataracts and dry eye syndrome. After careful review of scientific studies, my colleague Dr. Pelletier and I have determined the most important nutrients for the prevention of eye disease and the promotion of eye health. Each of these eye nutrients may decrease the risk of eye disease, either on its own or in conjunction with other nutrients.

In my optometric practice, my patients often have questions about the use of foods, vitamins, minerals and supplements to promote eye health. Most people have heard that antioxidants are important for healthy eyes. Some are aware of the eye health benefits of specific nutrients, such as beta-carotene. However, the majority of my patients are unsure about how to use this information when it comes to adding the nutrients to their diets.

In this section, I'll introduce all of the important eye nutrients, to give you the foundation for an understanding of how to incorporate them into an eye-healthy lifestyle that will develop further as you continue reading this book.

An Overview of Eye Nutrients

Nutrient	Type of Nutrient	Common Food Sources
Beta-carotene	Carotenoid	Fruits and vegetables
Lutein and zeaxanthin	Carotenoid	Fruits and vegetables, eggs
Vitamin C	Antioxidant	Fruits and vegetables
Vitamin D	Antioxidant	Fortified milk, fortified cereal flour
Vitamin E	Antioxidant	Oils, nuts, eggs, some fruits and vegetables
Zinc	Essential mineral	Seafood, meat, nuts, whole grains, fortified breakfast cereals
Fiber	Plant compound	Whole grains, fruits and vegetables
Omega-3 fatty acids	Essential fatty acids	Cold-water fish, some plant oils

FAQs

Q. What are antioxidants?

A. Antioxidants are a class of substances that help prevent oxidation in the body. They include vitamins (such as vitamins C, D and E), minerals (such as selenium) and phytonutrients (such as the carotenoids lutein and zeaxanthin).

- **Antioxidants and eye health:** Antioxidants may reduce the risk of AMD and cataracts.
- **Antioxidants and general health:** Antioxidants have been shown to reduce the risk of cardiovascular disease, respiratory disease and cancer. They can also enhance immune function.

Q. What is oxidation?

A. Oxidation is a chemical reaction within the body that changes a stable molecule into a free radical. Exposure to certain environmental factors, including ultraviolet light, hazardous chemicals and air pollution, causes free radicals to form. The natural aging process, poor dietary habits and smoking also trigger their formation. If left unchecked, free radicals will damage body tissues and can lead to a variety of chronic and age-related diseases, such as AMD, cancer and cardiovascular disease.

Q. What are carotenoids?

A. Carotenoids are pigments that give plants their color. There are more than 600 carotenoids in nature, 50 in the food chain and 15 in our bodies. Lutein, a carotenoid that is important for eye health, is also responsible for the bright yellow color of the marigold flower.

Of all the carotenoids, the most important to the human body are beta-carotene, lutein, zeaxanthin, lycopene, alpha-carotene and beta-cryptoxanthin. Carotenoids have been shown to act as antioxidants in the body. Specific carotenoids can also serve additional functions, such as filtering light or being converted into vitamin A.

Beta-Carotene

Beta-carotene is a carotenoid of orange color found in fruits and vegetables such as cantaloupe, apricots, squash, carrots and sweet potatoes. The body converts beta-carotene into vitamin A.

DIETARY REFERENCE INTAKES
- **RDA:** To date, no RDA for beta-carotene has been set; however, the Institute of Medicine recommends regular consumption of carotenoid-rich fruits and vegetables
- **UL:** To date, no UL for beta-carotene has been set

BETA-CAROTENE AND EYE HEALTH
Beta-carotene from food is important for eye health because the body converts it into vitamin A, which is used by the retina to create the vision signal.

BETA-CAROTENE AND GENERAL HEALTH

Higher blood levels of beta-carotene may decrease the risk of chronic disease. Beta-carotene has been shown to act as an antioxidant.

BE AWARE

Beta-carotene should not be taken in supplement form for the prevention of AMD for two reasons: safety and competition.

1. **Safety:** Smokers and recent ex-smokers who take beta-carotene supplements may have a higher risk of lung cancer.

2. **Competition:** When taken with lutein and zeaxanthin, beta-carotene supplements compete with those nutrients for uptake by the body, decreasing the absorption of lutein and zeaxanthin. Most people obtain an adequate amount of beta-carotene from food sources, while lutein and zeaxanthin intake from diet remains low.

Lutein and Zeaxanthin

Lutein and zeaxanthin are pigments that are abundant in the macula (the central part of the retina). The body cannot make lutein; therefore, we must obtain it from our diet. The body can convert lutein into a form of zeaxanthin called meso-zeaxanthin. It is thought that this conversion occurs when there are insufficient amounts of zeaxanthin in the eye.

In the eye, lutein and zeaxanthin absorb blue and ultraviolet light, protecting the macula from their harmful effects. Consuming lutein and zeaxanthin, either in foods or in a supplement, increases carotenoids in the macula.

Lutein and zeaxanthin are abundant in fruits and vegetables. Lutein is found in leafy green vegetables and egg yolks, zeaxanthin in orange bell peppers. Adding oil or other fats to foods high in lutein significantly increases your body's absorption of lutein.

DIETARY REFERENCE INTAKES

- **RDA:** To date, no RDA for lutein or zeaxanthin has been set; however, the Institute of Medicine recommends regular consumption of carotenoid-rich fruits and vegetables
- **UL:** To date, no UL for lutein or zeaxanthin has been set

LUTEIN AND ZEAXANTHIN AND EYE HEALTH

Scientific research shows that lutein can improve visual function in people with AMD. A high dietary intake of lutein and zeaxanthin has consistently been shown to protect against AMD and cataracts. A large randomized controlled trial (AREDS 2) demonstrated that people with moderate AMD who took lutein and zeaxanthin in supplement form along with other antioxidants (vitamin E, vitamin C and zinc) were less likely to progress to advanced AMD.

LUTEIN AND ZEAXANTHIN AND GENERAL HEALTH

Lutein and zeaxanthin are found in the skin and can help maintain healthy skin. They may also protect against cardiovascular disease and breast cancer. They are even found in the brain, and early studies are showing that lutein and zeaxanthin may be related to cognitive function.

> Lutein and zeaxanthin are found in our eyes, brain, skin and breast tissue.

Meso-Zeaxanthin

Meso-zeaxanthin is a pigment that the body makes from lutein. It is found exclusively in the eye and not in other parts of the body. It is not considered a dietary carotenoid, as it is not commonly found in food; however, it does appear in small amounts in shrimp shells, fish skin and some eggs from Mexico. Scientists are exploring whether supplementation with meso-zeaxanthin, in addition to lutein and zeaxanthin, may be beneficial in prevention of AMD.

Macular Pigment

Macular pigment is made up of lutein, zeaxanthin and meso-zeaxanthin. It absorbs blue wavelength light and acts as an antioxidant, protecting the rods and cones of the eye from oxidative damage. It is believed that macular pigment has two main purposes in the eye: to prevent damage to macular cells and to improve the macula's optical performance.

Macular Pigment and Vision

Macular pigment may help to increase contrast sensitivity, our ability to distinguish things when there is little difference between the image and the background. For example, reading very light gray print on white paper would require good contrast sensitivity. One way macular pigment might help with contrast sensitivity is by decreasing glare when we drive at night.

Macular Pigment and Disease Prevention

Macular pigment may help decrease your risk of developing AMD. In addition, the amount of macular pigment in the eye may correlate with the amount of lutein and zeaxanthin in the brain. Scientists believe that lutein and zeaxanthin may play a role in brain health and cognitive function; however, their exact role in brain health is not yet known.

Measuring Your Macular Pigment

Low macular pigment optical density may increase your risk of developing AMD. Ask your eye doctor for more information about having your macular pigment optical density measured, and for ways to minimize your risk for ocular disease and achieve your best vision. If you have low macular pigment, you may be able to increase it through diet and supplements.

Vitamin C

Vitamin C, also called ascorbic acid, is a water-soluble antioxidant found in fruits and vegetables. It is found in every structure of the eye. In fact, the amount of vitamin C in the aqueous humor of the eye is 10 to 20 times more than in the blood serum.

Vitamin C cannot be made or stored by the body, so it is essential to consume foods high in vitamin C several times per day. These include kiwifruit, raw bell peppers, raw broccoli, citrus fruits and leafy green vegetables.

DIETARY REFERENCE INTAKES
- **RDA:** Adult women, 75 mg/day; adult men, 90 mg/day
- **UL:** 2,000 mg/day for all adults

VITAMIN C AND EYE HEALTH
Diets high in vitamin C and other antioxidants have been shown to decrease the risk of AMD in elderly persons. Vitamin C can also decrease the risk of cataracts.

VITAMIN C AND GENERAL HEALTH
Vitamin C helps the body maintain a healthy immune system and increases its ability to absorb iron from plant foods. It may decrease the risk for stroke, heart attack and lung cancer.

BE AWARE
- High doses of vitamin C (more than 2,000 milligrams per day) may worsen symptoms in people prone to kidney stones.
- Taking more than 2,000 milligrams per day of vitamin C can cause diarrhea, nausea, stomach cramping, excess urination and skin rashes.

Vitamin D

Vitamin D is a fat-soluble vitamin stored by the body. Because the natural levels of vitamin D in foods are quite low, many foods, such as milk and cereal flour, are fortified with it. The body receives the majority of its vitamin D when UVB rays contact exposed skin, causing a chemical reaction that creates vitamin D. Less vitamin D is synthesized on cloudy days and during the winter. Wearing sunscreen with an SPF of 8 or higher also limits vitamin D production.

DIETARY REFERENCE INTAKES
- **AI:** Adults 19–50, 200 IU/day; adults 51–69, 400 IU/day; adults 70+, 600 IU/day
- **UL:** 2,000 IU/day for all adults

FAQ

Q. Should I take nutrient supplements, or is it better to try to get an adequate nutrient intake from my diet?

A. People with certain ocular and medical conditions, or risk factors for certain diseases, are not able to meet the nutritional requirements necessary for disease prevention (or progression prevention) through diet alone. It is important to take a supplement if a health care professional advises you to do so. However, a supplement is not a replacement for a healthy diet. The synergy of nutrients in whole foods has beneficial effects on our bodies that supplements cannot replicate.

You should make the decision to take a supplement only after you have had a discussion with your eye care provider. Pregnant women, breastfeeding women and people with health conditions must check with a physician before taking a supplement. Some supplements can interact with certain prescription and over-the-counter medications, causing adverse side effects or altering the efficacy of the medication. For this reason, it is important to inform your health care providers of all the prescription and nonprescription drugs and supplements you are taking.

VITAMIN D AND EYE HEALTH

Vitamin D may be associated with a decreased risk for early AMD.

VITAMIN D AND GENERAL HEALTH

Insufficient levels of vitamin D may increase the risk for osteoporosis by limiting calcium absorption in the body. In children, a lack of vitamin D, calcium or phosphate can lead to a disease called rickets, which causes weak bones, bone fractures, bowed legs and stunted growth. A sufficient vitamin D intake may decrease the risk for certain cancers, heart disease and type 2 diabetes.

BE AWARE

Vitamin D supplements may interact with certain medications, such as corticosteroids and cholesterol-lowering drugs.

DID YOU KNOW?

Winter Sun

From November to February in northern climates such as the northern states and Canada, sun exposure alone cannot provide adequate vitamin D. The angle of the sun is such that UVB rays are limited, so even on a sunny day there will be no vitamin D production.

Vitamin E

Vitamin E is a fat-soluble antioxidant found in oils, nuts, eggs and some fruits and vegetables, and in fortified cereals. Scientific studies show that vitamin E obtained from food may be more beneficial than vitamin E from supplements.

DIETARY REFERENCE INTAKES

- **RDA:** 15 mg/day for all adults
- **UL:** 1,000 mg/day for all adults

VITAMIN E AND EYE HEALTH

When taken with other antioxidants, vitamin E may decrease the risk of cataracts and AMD.

VITAMIN E AND GENERAL HEALTH

Vitamin E has been shown to protect the body against cancer and cardiovascular disease. It also works with vitamin C to boost the immune system.

BE AWARE

Take vitamin E supplements only under supervision by your doctor. One study suggests that taking daily high-dose supplements of 400 IU (about 360 mg) or more of vitamin E increases the risk of death in certain people. However, at lower doses, from diet or supplements, vitamin E is not harmful.

Zinc

Zinc is an essential trace mineral that exists in every cell of the body. It is found in seafood, meat, nuts, beans, whole grains and fortified breakfast cereals. Oysters are the best food source of zinc, but North Americans get most of their zinc from red meat and poultry.

DIETARY REFERENCE INTAKES

- **RDA:** Adult women, 8 mg/day; adult men, 11 mg/day
- **UL:** 40 mg/day for all adults

ZINC AND EYE HEALTH

Zinc intake from diet and supplements has been shown to protect against AMD.

ZINC AND GENERAL HEALTH

Zinc supports the immune system and the healing process, and it encourages normal growth and development during pregnancy, childhood and adolescence.

BE AWARE

Zinc toxicity occurs at 150 to 450 mg/day and can adversely affect the body's immune system, iron status, copper status and HDL ("good") cholesterol levels. This pertains only to zinc obtained through supplements; there is no evidence of adverse effects from zinc found naturally in foods.

Pro Tip

Zinc lozenges may decrease the duration of common cold symptoms.

Fiber

Dietary fiber is the portion of plant foods that the body is unable to digest. It exists in two forms: soluble fiber and insoluble fiber. Diets high in fiber support a healthy digestive system.

- **Sources of soluble fiber:** Barley, beans, citrus fruits, oat bran, oatmeal, strawberries
- **Sources of insoluble fiber:** Brussels sprouts, cabbage, carrots, cereal, whole wheat bread

DIETARY REFERENCE INTAKES
- **AI:** Adult women, 21–25 g/day; adult men, 30–38 g/day
- **UL:** To date, no UL for fiber has been set

FIBER AND EYE HEALTH
Diets with a high glycemic index can increase the risk of AMD and cataracts. Plant foods high in fiber tend to have a low glycemic index, so a diet rich in these foods is beneficial to eye health.

FIBER AND GENERAL HEALTH
When eaten as part of a heart-friendly diet, soluble fiber can decrease blood cholesterol. Insoluble fiber helps maintain healthy bowels.

> The American Heart Association and the Canadian Heart and Stroke Foundation recommend a diet high in fiber. Supporting a healthy cardio-vascular system also promotes healthy eyes.

Omega-3 Fatty Acids

Three important omega-3 fatty acids are DHA (docosahexaenoic acid), EPA (eicosapentaenoic acid) and ALA (alpha-linolenic acid). DHA and EPA are found in fish oils; ALA is found in nuts, flax seeds and vegetable oils.

DHA and EPA help decrease inflammation in the body. The body converts ALA into DHA and EPA, but because it is not an efficient process, DHA and EPA are best consumed directly. However, ALA does have beneficial effects of its own and should still be included in a healthy diet.

Sources of Omega-3 Fatty Acids

Omega-3 Fatty Acid	Food Sources
ALA	Avocados, canola oil, flax seeds and flaxseed oil, soy products, walnuts and walnut oil, wheat germ and wheat germ oil
DHA and EPA	Cold-water fish, especially salmon, sardines, rainbow trout and mackerel

DIETARY REFERENCE INTAKES
- **AI:** Adult women, 1.1 g/day; adult men, 1.6 g/day
- **UL:** To date, no UL for omega-3 fatty acids has been set

OMEGA-3 FATTY ACIDS AND EYE HEALTH
Consumption of fish high in omega-3 fatty acids can decrease the risk of AMD. Both fish oils (DHA and EPA) and flaxseed oil (ALA) are therapeutic for patients with dry eye syndrome.

OMEGA-3 FATTY ACIDS AND GENERAL HEALTH
The American Heart Association recommends eating cold-water fish at least twice a week, and suggests that foods high in ALA should be included in a healthy diet. Fish oil has been proven to reduce the risk and severity of heart disease, high cholesterol, rheumatoid arthritis and dementia.

BE AWARE
- Certain fish and fish oils contain high levels of mercury. The USDA recommends that women who are or may become pregnant, as well as breastfeeding women, eat only 8 to 10 ounces (250 to 300 g) of fish or shellfish per week. Health Canada recommends that women consume 5 ounces (150 g) of fish per week during pregnancy, with a focus on fish with low methylmercury levels. For a complete list of good fish choices, see page 24 of the "Dietary Guidelines for Americans."
- The USDA and Health Canada recommend that pregnant women, women who may become pregnant and breastfeeding women avoid eating shark, swordfish and king mackerel because of their high mercury content.
- Do not take more than 3 grams of omega-3 fatty acids per day unless under the care of a physician. High levels may cause excessive bleeding in rare cases.

Omega-6:Omega-3 Ratio

Omega-6 fatty acids are pro-inflammatory, while omega-3 fatty acids are anti-inflammatory. Our bodies require this opposition, but in the right proportion. Humans are thought to have evolved by eating a diet that provided equal amounts of omega-6 and omega-3 fatty acids (a 1:1 ratio). In our ancestors' diets, substantial amounts of omega-3 fatty acids were found in wild plants and wild game. Many natural sources of omega-3 fatty acids are now depleted, resulting in a change in our dietary ratios. In our current diets, omega-6 fatty acids are generally consumed over omega-3 fatty acids at a ratio of 14:1.

Consuming a greater proportion of omega-6 fatty acids results in the body remaining in an inflammatory state. We do need the pro-inflammatory component of the omega-6s to heal from injuries, but once the healing phase is done, we need the anti-inflammatory effects of the omega-3s to return to a balanced state. Since the typical North American consumes many omega-6 fatty acids and far fewer omega-3 fatty acids, we need to focus on ways to balance the proportion by increasing our omega-3 fatty acid intake.

Chapter 5
Eyefoods

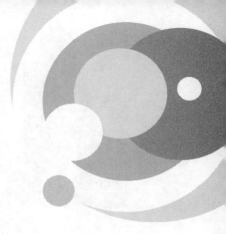

A diet filled with the right foods helps to preserve eye health and fight eye disease. After reviewing the nutrient content of hundreds of whole foods, my colleague Dr. Pelletier and I selected the foods best suited to the promotion of healthy eyes, based on the amount and variety of eye nutrients they contain. We call these foods "eyefoods."

Eyefoods are loaded with nutrients that are beneficial to eye health. To obtain the greatest benefit, you should include as many eyefoods in your diet as possible. An eyefood-rich diet will help you maintain your vision and prevent eye disease while also decreasing your risk for cardiovascular disease and many types of cancer.

In this chapter, I will describe the eyefoods and outline how each food promotes eye health and helps prevent eye disease. I will suggest a target for how much of each food to eat and provide tips on how to integrate eyefoods into daily meals for yourself and your family.

> *An eyefood-rich diet will help you maintain your vision and prevent eye disease while also decreasing your risk for cardiovascular disease and many types of cancer.*

Leafy Green Vegetables

Leafy green vegetables are the gold medalists of eyefoods, as they contain all of the essential nutrients necessary for healthy eyes. Raw and cooked leafy green vegetables provide different nutritional benefits. When you eat raw leafy green vegetables, your body absorbs more vitamin C, as cooking food typically decreases vitamin C content. However, when you eat cooked leafy greens, your body absorbs more lutein and zeaxanthin. In fact, although cooking these carotenoids may decrease their content in the food, it seems to increase their bioavailabity (your body's ability to absorb the nutrients in food).

To get the most out of the foods in this category, eat a wide variety of leafy greens, as each type contains vital nutrients to nourish your body and your eyes. Try sampling all of the different options, and enjoy them both raw and cooked.

EYEFOODS
Arugula, Chinese broccoli, collard greens, dandelion greens, kale, leaf lettuce, napa cabbage, pea shoots, radicchio, rapini, romaine lettuce, spinach, Swiss chard, watercress

TOP EYEFOODS

Kale, spinach, dandelion greens

EYE NUTRIENTS

Beta-carotene, fiber, lutein and zeaxanthin, omega-3 fatty acids, vitamin C, vitamin E, zinc

WEEKLY TARGETS

- **Raw:** 1 cup (250 mL) or 1 large handful, seven times a week
- **Cooked:** ½ cup (125 mL), twice a week

BE AWARE

People on blood thinners must watch their intake of leafy green vegetables. Blood thinners work by decreasing the activity of vitamin K, which is abundant in leafy greens. Too many leafy green vegetables in a person's diet can decrease the efficacy of blood thinner medications and cause serious complications. If you take blood thinners, discuss any potential changes in your diet with your physician.

Kale

This curly cruciferous vegetable is the number one food in the leafy greens category. It is a cold-weather vegetable that grows best in the spring and fall. It has a smoother flavor when harvested after the first frost.

Kale contains three times as much lutein and zeaxanthin as dandelion greens and spinach. If you eat just one medium leaf of raw kale a day, you get enough lutein and zeaxanthin to meet the eyefoods daily target.

Enjoy kale both raw and cooked (see Mix-and-Match Sautéed Greens, page 176). Kale also makes a great substitute for cabbage in dishes such as cabbage rolls.

Spinach

Spinach and baby spinach are becoming more commonplace in the North American diet. We have known the health benefits of spinach for years: think of Popeye's bulging muscles as he consumed a can of these powerful greens in the old Saturday morning cartoons.

Dandelion Greens

Don't let its name scare you — this is indeed a gem of a leafy green vegetable. It's widely enjoyed as a cooked side dish in Mediterranean countries, and a handful of raw dandelion greens added to a salad with leaf or romaine lettuce adds wonderful texture and a peppery flavor.

Unlike kale, which is harvested in the fall or winter, dandelion greens are harvested in early spring (even before asparagus).

Arugula

This peppery, slightly bitter lettuce is also known as rocket. It is common in Mediterranean cuisine and tastes great in salads, omelets and stir-fries or as a pizza topping.

Chinese Broccoli

Gai lan, as Chinese broccoli is called in Cantonese, is part of the broccoli family, but this delicious green is longer and leaner than regular broccoli and has a sharper flavor. It is common in Chinese, Vietnamese and Thai cuisine. Enjoy it stir-fried or steamed with ginger.

Collard Greens

Collard greens are commonly found in diets in the southern United States. They are thought to have first been cultivated by the Ancient Greeks. They are part of the cabbage family and have a slightly bitter flavor.

Leaf Lettuce

This tender, lighter lettuce comes in green and red varieties. Because it tends to be softer than other lettuces, when using it in salads, be sure to add dressing just before eating. If you dress the salad too soon, the lettuce gets soggy.

Napa Cabbage

Also known as Chinese cabbage, napa cabbage is pale green, has ruffled leaves and tastes great raw in slaws and salads. It is also a great addition to stir-fries and tastes wonderful when grilled with olive oil. In Korean cuisine, it is an ingredient in kimchi, a fermented side dish.

Pea Shoots

These delicate shoots are harvested 2 to 4 weeks after seeding. The nutrients are concentrated in the delicate leaves, which are a great source of lutein. They have an intense pea flavor and both the stems and leaves are edible. Use them in a salad, add them to a stir-fry or toss them into soup just before serving.

Radicchio

Radicchio, also known as Italian chicory, originated in the Veneto region of Northern Italy. It is a late-season winter vegetable that tastes great in salads or grilled with olive oil. I can hear you saying, "But radicchio isn't green!" Indeed, many common varieties aren't green; nevertheless, radicchio's lutein content is similar to that of other leafy greens, so it fits into this category despite its color.

Rapini

Rapini, or broccoli rabe, is common in Italian cuisine and is a distant relative to the turnip. It has an earthy, peppery taste and tastes great with whole-grain pasta.

Romaine Lettuce

A popular lettuce in Caesar salads, romaine has a crisp texture and a sweet flavor. Most supermarkets carry whole heads of romaine and packages of romaine hearts, which tend to be crunchier than the outer leaves.

Swiss Chard

Swiss chard's large leaves can be green or red. When enjoyed raw, it has a slightly bitter flavor. When cooked, the bitterness fades and the flavor becomes sweeter.

Watercress

This leafy green is crisp and spicy, with a hint of pepper. It tastes like you are biting into a radish. Watercress tastes great in salads, wraps and soups, and makes a delicious addition to scrambled eggs. In England, it is often served in sandwiches as part of high tea.

Eyefoods Tips: Leafy Greens

- Try to incorporate at least two types of leafy green vegetables into your diet most days. For example, make a salad for two people with a handful of baby spinach and one of romaine hearts. The crispness of the romaine hearts will balance the smooth texture of the spinach.
- If your palate is not accustomed to the tastes and textures of leafy green vegetables, start slowly. Romaine and leaf lettuce should please any palate, but it may take time to enjoy the more intense flavors of kale, radicchio and arugula. Add a couple of leaves, cut into bite-size pieces, to any salad. Don't be surprised if you come to love the intensity of their flavor.
- Add extra virgin olive oil, canola oil or walnut oil to cooked or raw leafy greens, to increase the body's absorption of lutein.
- Every week, buy one bunch of any leafy green vegetable per family of four.
- For quick and easy meal preparation, store washed, chopped and blanched greens in the freezer.
- It takes 8 cups (2 L) of raw leafy greens to make 1 cup (250 mL) of cooked greens.

Cold-Water Fish

Scientists have found that eating cold-water fish (also known as fatty fish) has protective effects against age-related macular degeneration (AMD), cataracts and dry eye syndrome. The omega-3 fatty acids found in these fish may also decrease the risk of certain chronic diseases, such as cardiovascular disease and cancer.

The health benefits of fish make it an important addition to every diet. However, not all fish is created equal. Most fish are a great source of lean protein, but for the benefits of omega-3 fatty acids, some fish are a better choice than others. Salmon is a top eyefood because it has a high amount of omega-3 fatty acids. Other good sources include sardines, tuna and mackerel.

EYEFOODS
Arctic char, mackerel, herring, rainbow trout, salmon, sardines, tuna

TOP EYEFOODS
Salmon, sardines, tuna

EYE NUTRIENTS
Omega-3 fatty acids (DHA and EPA), vitamin D (in sardines), vitamin E

WEEKLY TARGETS
- **Salmon:** $3\frac{1}{2}$ oz (100 g) cooked, twice a week
- **Other cold-water fish:** $3\frac{1}{2}$ oz (100 g) cooked, twice a week

BE AWARE
- Certain fish and fish oils contain high levels of mercury. The United States Department of Agriculture (USDA) recommends that women who are or may become pregnant, as well as breastfeeding women, eat only 8 to 10 ounces

> **DID YOU KNOW?**
> ....
> **Fish and Life Expectancy**
>
> Fish is abundant in Mediterranean and Asian cuisines, and it has important benefits for the cardiovascular system and the brain. Cultures in which people have a long life expectancy and lower rates of chronic diseases often include fish as a dietary staple.

(250 to 300 g) of fish or shellfish per week. Health Canada recommends that women consume 5 ounces (150 grams) of fish per week during pregnancy, with a focus on fish with low methylmercury levels. For a complete list of good fish choices, see page 24 of the "Dietary Guidelines for Americans."

- The USDA and Health Canada recommend that pregnant women, women who may become pregnant and breastfeeding women avoid eating shark, swordfish and king mackerel because of their high mercury content.

Salmon

Salmon has a wonderfully rich texture and flavor. Choose either wild salmon or high-quality farmed salmon, which have lower levels of mercury and higher amounts of omega-3 fatty acids. Ask your fishmonger where your fish is sourced, then visit seafood.edf.org to determine the mercury level of the salmon.

Sardines

Some say sardines are one of the healthiest foods around. They're packed with omega-3 fatty acids, vitamin E and vitamin D. As an added bonus, they are inexpensive and readily available in almost every supermarket. Sardines are popping up on the menus of the best restaurants, as their image is changing from a simple staple to more gourmet fare. In Mediterranean countries, it is common to find fresh sardines, though in North America, most sardines are canned. Sardines can sometimes be found in the freezer section of the supermarket. Try grilling them from frozen.

Meal and Snack Ideas

- Brush salmon fillets with olive oil, season with sea salt and black pepper, and bake at 375°F (190°C) for 15 to 20 minutes or until fish is opaque and flakes easily when tested with a fork. Serve with sautéed or steamed leafy green vegetables.
- Make a high-protein salad with a can of boneless sardines, orange bell peppers and sun-dried tomatoes.
- Create an attractive pepper boat by cutting an orange, yellow or red bell pepper in half and filling it with tuna salad.
- On a sheet of foil, layer rainbow trout on top of a bed of thinly sliced lemons, onions and parsley. Season with avocado oil, sea salt and pepper, then fold the foil into an enclosed packet. Grill on medium-high heat for 15 to 20 minutes or until fish flakes easily when tested with a fork.

How Clean Is Your Fish?

Fish are an important part of a healthy diet. They contain the omega-3 fatty acids DHA and EPA, which help maintain eye health, cardiovascular health and cognitive health and decrease inflammation in the body. The nutrients in fish also support growth and development, so eating fish is particularly important for children and pregnant women.

Most North Americans do not get enough omega-3 fatty acids in their diet. To help prevent the onset of chronic eye diseases, such as AMD and dry eye syndrome, the Eyefoods Plan recommends eating cold-water fish four times per week.

As important as it is to eat more fish, there are real concerns about the contamination and sustainability of the fish available to us. To keep both your family and the oceans healthy, ask these two questions before you go shopping for fish:

1. Is this fish contaminated?
2. Is this fish sustainable?

Is This Fish Contaminated?

Two contaminants of concern in fish are mercury and PCBs (polychlorinated biphenyls).

One of the reasons mercury is hazardous to health is that it enters our cells effortlessly and interferes with the body's normal functioning. It also crosses the placenta of mammals and can interfere with normal fetal development.

How does mercury get into fish? Human-generated mercury enters the atmosphere mostly from industry, especially coal-burning plants. It is a global issue, as air currents carry mercury across the planet. When mercury falls into the ocean, it is converted to methylmercury and is absorbed by living things, beginning with plankton. It then accumulates more with each rung of the food chain. Small fish are lower on the food chain than large fish, so they have lower amounts of mercury. The bigger the fish, the more mercury.

Although dangerous to our health, mercury can be eliminated from our bodies over time. However, in cases of long-term mercury exposure, it can take up to a year to fully eliminate it.

PCBs are manmade chemicals that were used in industry before being banned in the 1970s. PCBs are slow to break down and may still be a concern in certain fish.

For more information on contaminants in fish, visit safinacenter.org/issues/mercury-seafood or http://seafood.edf.org/pcbs-fish-and-shellfish?.

Is This Fish Sustainable?

Oceans cover nearly 75% of the Earth's surface and are vital to maintaining life and our climate. Overfishing has a major impact on the marine ecosystem and the sustainability of many marine species. Industrial fishing, which uses large, mechanized vessels to find and catch fish, has led to the decline of many fish species. Coastal development, pollution and climate change also affect the marine environment.

Science-based catch limits and better management of industrialized fisheries give us hope in turning the tide on overfishing. Many fisheries in Alaska are currently using these principles.

Aquaculture, or fish farming, has the potential to provide a solution for the ecological impact of industrialized fishing, but it has its own set of problems. First off, many types of fish eat other species of fish, so wild fish are needed to feed the farmed fish. Second, pollution is often an issue when fish are farmed in contained areas. Certain types of farmed fish are recommended, while others are best avoided.

For more information on sustainable seafood choices, see the recommendations at Monterey Bay Aquarium Seafood Watch: www.seafoodwatch.org/seafood-recommendations.

Tuna

Canned tuna is a staple in almost every pantry in North America. It is a convenient way to add fish to a busy lifestyle. Unfortunately, there are concerns over the mercury content in canned tuna. The USDA and Health Canada recommend choosing canned light tuna over albacore (white) tuna because of its lower mercury content.

Eyefoods Tips: Cold-Water Fish

- Buy 10 ounces (300 g) of skinless salmon per family member per week. Bake it all at once for dinner and use the leftovers to make a salmon salad to enjoy in sandwiches the next day.
- Give yourself a chance to develop a taste for sardines and mackerel by trying them every so often. Soon you will find yourself reaching for them!
- Keep a variety of canned sardines and mackerel handy for an easy lunch. You can get boneless skinless sardines and mackerel in different delicious sauces. Try a mustard flavor for a quick and tasty sandwich.
- If you find it difficult to prepare fish at home, order grilled or baked fish when dining out.

Orange Vegetables

Orange vegetables are the beta-carotene stars of the eyefoods. These brightly colored gems provide a bigger boost of beta-carotene than any other food group, along with significant amounts of most other eye nutrients. In addition to preventing eye disease, the antioxidants in these foods help to protect the body from diseases caused by oxidative damage, such as heart disease and cancer.

An eye-friendly diet includes many foods rich in beta-carotene. Eating a variety of orange vegetables will ensure that you receive their maximum nutritional benefits.

• CAUTION •

Research shows that beta-carotene supplements can increase the risk of lung cancer in people who smoke or who recently quit.

EYEFOODS
Acorn squash, buttercup squash, butternut squash, carrots, pumpkin, spaghetti squash, sweet potatoes

TOP EYEFOOD
Sweet potatoes

EYE NUTRIENTS
Beta-carotene, fiber, lutein and zeaxanthin, vitamin C, vitamin E, zinc

- **Cooked orange vegetables:** $1/2$ cup (125 mL), three times a week
- **Raw carrots:** $1/2$ cup (125 mL), three times a week

Sweet Potatoes

Sweet potatoes top the list as the number one orange vegetable because they are the best food source of beta-carotene. They also contain a significant amount of fiber. They are readily available throughout the year in supermarkets.

Carrots

Perhaps the best-known eyefood, carrots are inexpensive, versatile and make a great snack. Drinking carrot juice is a great way to get a beta-carotene blast, but enjoy it in moderation — consuming too much can cause your skin to appear orange (see sidebar, page 76).

Winter Squash

There are many different types of winter squash. Butternut, buttercup, acorn and spaghetti squash are all great choices. In addition, canned pumpkin purée is a convenient, healthy pantry staple. Be sure to buy 100% canned pumpkin and not pumpkin pie filling, which contains added sugar.

Pro Tip

Try eating the skin of the sweet potato — it is loaded with vital nutrients and fiber.

DID YOU KNOW?

Buy Local

Sweet potatoes, carrots and winter squash are abundant in late summer and fall at local farmers' markets. These root vegetables store for weeks in a cool, dry place.

Meal and Snack Ideas

- Enjoy baby carrots as a snack with hummus or white bean dip.
- Sweet potatoes make a great substitution for white potatoes. Enjoy them baked, roasted or mashed with a splash of extra virgin olive oil and a sprinkle of salt and pepper.
- Cut a butternut squash in half, roast it and drizzle with maple syrup.
- Create delicious fall soups with any orange vegetable superstar. Top with crushed walnuts.

Eyefoods Tips: Orange Vegetables

- Eat at least two different types of orange vegetables per week.
- Keep carrots in the refrigerator so they are always available for a quick snack.
- Keep frozen butternut squash in the freezer for a quick side dish to turkey or fish.
- Make canned pumpkin a staple in your pantry and add it to soups, stews and muffins.
- Make a beautiful centerpiece for your kitchen table or island with a variety of winter squash. They will be readily available to roast and enjoy.

Orange Bell Peppers

Of all the bell peppers, orange peppers have the highest amount of eye-healthy nutrients. They are an excellent source of zeaxanthin, the macular pigment that acts as a sidekick to lutein. As we now know, lutein and zeaxanthin may reduce the risk of AMD and cataracts. In addition, just half an orange pepper contains more than 50% of the daily eyefoods target of vitamin C, making them the number one source of this essential nutrient. They also offer higher levels of vitamin E than other vegetables, so they are an excellent low-calorie source of that vitamin, which is more commonly obtained from oils and other fats.

Orange bell peppers have just the right mix of nutrients to make them an eyefood on their own, but yellow, red and green peppers also contain high amounts of vitamin C. Enjoy bell peppers of all colors, but fill your shopping cart with more orange peppers to get the most eye nutrients.

EYE NUTRIENTS

Beta-carotene, lutein and zeaxanthin, vitamin C, vitamin E

WEEKLY TARGET

- ½ pepper, four times a week (2 servings raw, 2 servings cooked)

Meal and Snack Ideas

- Enjoy raw orange pepper strips as a snack or as part of a vegetable plate.
- Add chopped orange peppers to a spinach or bean salad.
- Cut an orange pepper in half or into quarters to make a pepper boat. Fill it with egg, tuna or turkey salad for a healthy lunch.
- Sauté orange, red and yellow pepper strips with boneless skinless turkey breast strips as a filling for a whole wheat pita or tortilla.

Eyefoods Tips: Orange Bell Peppers

- Eat two orange peppers, one raw and one cooked, every week to increase your intake of zeaxanthin.
- Encourage your children to eat orange peppers like apples! They make a low-calorie, nutrient-dense snack.
- Keep sliced orange peppers in the fridge for a quick and easy snack during the day. Dip them in hummus for a protein boost.

Green Vegetables

There are a lot of green vegetables out there, but what the eyefoods options in this category have in common is that they are all high in lutein, zeaxanthin, vitamin C and fiber.

You can find fresh Brussels sprouts, broccoli and green beans throughout the year at the supermarket and locally grown in the late summer and early fall. Asparagus and green peas are harvested in late spring and early summer. Zucchini is abundant during the summer months. During the winter, select frozen vegetables over fresh. Fresh vegetables have to travel long distances to reach your supermarket in the winter, so their nutrient content will have decreased. Food processing companies freeze fruits and vegetables immediately after harvest, when nutrient quantities are at their peak, so frozen vegetables maintain the majority of their nutrients.

EYEFOODS

Asparagus, broccoli, Brussels sprouts, green beans, green peas, zucchini

EYE NUTRIENTS

Beta-carotene, fiber, lutein and zeaxanthin, vitamin C, vitamin E

WEEKLY TARGET

- **Raw or cooked:** $1/2$ cup (125 mL), seven times a week

Meal and Snack Ideas

- Use raw asparagus to make a spring salad. Thinly slice asparagus and toss with olive oil, balsamic vinegar, salt and pepper.
- Enjoy raw broccoli with white bean dip or hummus.
- Make a colorful salad with raw broccoli, dried apricots and walnuts.
- Steam Brussels sprouts or green beans with a drizzle of walnut oil or extra virgin olive oil and a sprinkle of sea salt.
- Thaw frozen peas for 20 minutes and add them to a green salad.
- Surprise your children with handfuls of half-thawed peas as a tide-me-over before dinner.
- Slice zucchini lengthwise, brush with avocado oil and grill over medium heat until grill marks appear and the zucchini softens. Enjoy throughout the week on salads.

Pro Tip

If you use canned vegetables, choose those without added salt whenever possible.

Eyefood Focus

Broccoli is particularly rich in vitamin C, though cooking decreases the amount available to your body. I recommend eating both raw and cooked broccoli every week.

Eyefood Focus

Zucchini is a source of lutein and can be enjoyed both raw and cooked.

Eyefoods Tips: Green Vegetables

- Buy two or three types of green vegetables each week to enjoy a variety at different meals.
- Gently steam enough green beans for two meals. Enjoy half the beans at one meal and use the rest in a salad or eat them as a snack within the next few days.
- Keep frozen peas handy for a nutritious last-minute side dish.

Eggs

An important eyefood, eggs contain significant amounts of vitamin E, lutein and the omega-3 fatty acids ALA (alpha-linolenic acid) and DHA (docosahexaenoic acid). Read labels and select the eggs that are highest in omega-3s, laid by chickens that have been fed a diet high in flax seeds and corn. Eggs that are high in omega-3s also tend to be a good source of vitamin E, and they contain a significant amount of lutein that is readily absorbed by our bodies.

Eaten in moderation, eggs provide the body with many healthful nutrients that ward off chronic disease and promote long-term eye health. Most of an egg's nutrients are in the yolk, so eat the entire egg for its full nutritional benefit.

EYE NUTRIENTS
Lutein and zeaxanthin, omega-3 fatty acids, vitamin E, zinc

WEEKLY TARGET
- 2 eggs, twice a week

BE AWARE
If you have heart disease or diabetes, or a family history of one of these conditions, consult your physician about appropriate egg consumption.

Meal and Snack Ideas

- Enjoy boiled eggs drizzled with olive oil and seasoned with salt and pepper on a slice of whole-grain toast for a nutritious breakfast or lunch.
- Make a delicious frittata or omelet with orange bell peppers and spinach.
- Serve bite-size portions of frittata as hors d'oeuvres.
- Try making sabayon, a classic French dessert prepared with egg yolks and topped with berries.

Eyefoods Tips: Eggs

- Eggs are both healthy and delicious when boiled, poached or scrambled, and they make a great meal as an omelet or frittata.
- To limit saturated fat and total fat intake, avoid cooking eggs in large amounts of butter or vegetable oil.
- If you enjoy egg salad as a quick lunch or snack, try using crispy romaine hearts or radicchio leaves in place of bread for an even more powerful lutein treat.

Fruit and Fruit Juice

Fruit and fruit juice are good sources of vitamin C. Since the body cannot store vitamin C, you should eat foods rich in it several times a day. Fruit is also full of other antioxidants that help to prevent disease, and enjoying a piece of fresh fruit can go a long way to satisfying a sweet tooth. Kiwifruit, cantaloupe and avocado are the top eyefoods, but eat a variety of fruits to experience the greatest synergy of nutrients.

EYEFOODS

Apricots, avocado (yes, it's a fruit!), berries, cantaloupe, citrus fruits, kiwifruit, other fruits

TOP EYEFOODS

Kiwifruit, cantaloupe, avocado

EYE NUTRIENTS

Beta-carotene, fiber, lutein and zeaxanthin, omega-3 fatty acids (avocado), vitamin C, vitamin E, zinc

DAILY TARGETS

- **Fruit:** Three servings per day
- **Fruit juice:** 1 cup (250 mL) of unsweetened fruit juice per day; 2 tablespoons (30 mL) of lemon juice per day

Pro Tip

If you are trying to lose weight or have diabetes, avoid fruit juice.

Kiwifruit

The highest fruit source of vitamin C, kiwifruit is the top eyefood in the fruit category. Kiwis taste best ripe, so select fruits that are soft to the touch.

Cantaloupe

High in beta-carotene, cantaloupe is a versatile fruit that can be enjoyed with low-fat yogurt for breakfast or as a tasty dessert.

Avocado

Although not sweet, avocado has a beautiful creamy, nutty flavor and is a source of the plant-based omega-3 fatty acid ALA, zinc, lutein, zeaxanthin and vitamin E. Avocados are high in calories, so limit your intake to half the fruit per serving.

A simple way to eat a kiwi is to cut it in half and scoop out the fruit with a teaspoon. You can also try eating the skin, as they do in New Zealand.

Fruit Juice

It is difficult to reach the daily eyefoods target for vitamin C by eating fruit alone. Adding 100% fruit juice to your diet helps increase vitamin C intake. However, even unsweetened fruit juice can be high in sugar and calories, so enjoy it in moderation. Good juice choices include orange juice, apple juice with added vitamin C and pineapple juice. Concord grape juice, pomegranate juice and low-sodium vegetable cocktail are other good options.

Meal and Snack Ideas

- Eat a kiwi each morning while you wait for your oatmeal or whole wheat toast to cook.
- Freeze sliced cantaloupe or kiwifruit when it is in season. Enjoy it slightly thawed as a refreshing after-dinner treat.
- Use a melon baller to create cantaloupe balls for an attractive fruit plate.
- Add half an avocado to a grilled vegetable sandwich.
- Treat yourself to avocado and crab salad on a whole wheat pita for lunch.

Eyefoods Tips: Fruit and Fruit Juice

- Start your day with fruit.
- Eat kiwifruit often — aim for one per day.
- Buy one cantaloupe every week for a family of four.
- Keep a jar of dried apricots on your counter and enjoy a few daily. Dried fruit is high in sugar, so limit your consumption to four pieces per day.
- Juice one lemon per person every day and dilute the juice in water, tea or another fruit juice, or sprinkle it over an avocado and crab salad.
- Create your own exciting juice combinations from leftover fresh fruit. You can find affordable, good-quality juicers at most department stores.
- Choose freshly squeezed or frozen orange juice whenever possible.
- Choose canned or bottled apple juice over frozen apple juice.

Lean Protein

Turkey breast and lean beef are important eyefoods because they contain large amounts of zinc and vitamin E. It is easier to achieve an optimal daily intake of zinc and vitamin E from your diet if you consume some lean meat, poultry, fish or seafood, but limit your consumption to no more than 6 ounces (175 g) of cooked meat per day. A $3\frac{1}{2}$-ounce (100 g) portion is approximately the size of a deck of playing cards.

EYEFOODS
Beef (lean cuts), canned crabmeat, chicken, clams, oysters, scallops, turkey (breast and dark meat)

EYE NUTRIENTS
Omega-3 fatty acids (DHA and EPA), zinc, vitamin E

WEEKLY TARGETS
- **Turkey breast:** $3^1/_2$ ounces (100 g) cooked meat, four times a week
- **Lean cuts of beef:** $3^1/_2$ ounces (100 g) cooked meat, twice a week

BE AWARE
It is difficult to achieve the RDA of zinc without consuming some meat or seafood. Vegetarians need to carefully monitor their zinc intake.

Pro Tip
Certain meats can be high in saturated fat, so choose leaner cuts, limit portion sizes and remove the skin from turkey and chicken.

Meal and Snack Ideas

- Make a sandwich with turkey breast, whole-grain bread, sliced apples, low-fat Swiss cheese and Dijon mustard. Grill in a panini press or on the stove. Drizzle with balsamic glaze.
- Make a stir-fry with lean beef and broccoli. Add reduced-sodium soy sauce, minced garlic and black pepper. Serve over barley or brown rice.
- Sprinkle canned crab over low-fat cream cheese and seafood sauce for a tasty dip. Enjoy with baby carrots or whole-grain pita toasts.

Eyefoods Tips: Lean Protein

- Use turkey breast fillets in place of chicken breasts. The zinc content is much greater in turkey than in chicken.
- Don't reserve turkey dinners for holidays. Roast a turkey for a great Sunday meal with lots of leftovers.
- Use ground turkey instead of ground beef for healthier burgers, meatballs and chili.
- Use canned crab as you would use canned tuna or salmon. Add it to salads and pastas, or use it to make a quick, flavorful dip.
- Eat cooked or smoked oysters occasionally. They are the top eyefood for zinc!

Nuts and Seeds

These nutrient-rich nibbles are powerful eyefoods that contain generous amounts of nutrients. Each nut and seed has its own nutritional benefits, so eat a good variety. To enjoy a healthy selection of nuts, simply prepare the Eyefoods Nut Mix (page 222) and eat a small handful (about 16 grams) per day. This nut mix contains a balanced amount of vitamin E, zinc and the omega-3 fatty acid ALA.

Unsalted raw or dry-roasted nuts and seeds are best. If you buy large quantities at a time, freeze them to prevent oxidation, which gives them a rancid taste and decreases their nutrient content. Many varieties of nuts and seeds are available in the bulk section of most supermarkets. Raw cashews and peanuts can be found at health food or bulk food stores.

> **Eyefood Focus**
>
> Eating nuts may protect against the progression of AMD, cardiovascular disease and type 2 diabetes.

EYEFOODS
Almonds, cashews, dry-roasted soybeans, hazelnuts, pecans, pine nuts, pistachios, pumpkin seeds, sunflower seeds, walnuts

TOP EYEFOODS
Almonds, walnuts, cashews, sunflower seeds, pumpkin seeds

Nut or Seed	Key Eye Nutrient
Almonds	Vitamin E
Walnuts	Omega-3 fatty acids (ALA)
Cashews	Zinc
Sunflower seeds	Vitamin E
Pumpkin seeds	Zinc

EYE NUTRIENTS
Fiber, omega-3 fatty acids (ALA), vitamin E, zinc

DAILY TARGET
- **Eyefoods Nut Mix:** 1 small handful per day

BE AWARE
Nuts and nut butters are high in calories, so consume only one handful of nuts or 2 tablespoons (30 mL) of nut butter per day. It's a good idea to reduce your fat intake from other sources when adding nuts to your diet. The best way to eliminate excess fat is to reduce your meat, butter or margarine intake.

DID YOU KNOW?

Nut Butters

Nutritious and tasty nut butters are a convenient way to enjoy the health benefits of nuts. Choose unsweetened natural peanut, almond or cashew butter. All are available in well-stocked supermarkets and health food stores.

Meal and Snack Ideas

- Add walnuts and almonds to brown rice for a creative side dish.
- Make homemade pesto by combining pine nuts, extra virgin olive oil, garlic and basil in a food processor or blender. Mix the pesto with whole wheat pasta or use it as a spread on whole wheat bread.
- Make a trail mix with dried apricots and a variety of nuts and seeds.
- Make a decadent hazelnut spread by mixing hazelnut butter with a little unsweetened cocoa powder, milk and honey.

Eyefoods Tips: Nuts and Seeds

- Eat nuts or seeds with your breakfast to include protein in the first meal of the day. The protein kick will delay midmorning hunger, which can lead to snacking on less-nutritious foods.
- Before adding them to a salad or rice bowl, toast nuts or seeds in a dry skillet for a few minutes to enhance their flavor.
- Buy fresh nuts in their shells in late fall and winter. Enjoy them with the family after dinner as a fun treat.

Whole Grains

Whole grains have a high fiber content and a low glycemic index. Current research shows that diets full of foods with a high glycemic index, such as white bread and sugar, can increase the risk of cataracts and AMD. As much as possible, choose whole-grain foods over refined carbohydrates such as white bread, rice or pasta. In fact, I recommend that you aim to eliminate refined grains from your diet entirely. Whole-grain bread, brown rice and whole-grain pasta are readily available in supermarkets, so it is merely a question of changing your habits.

Eating whole grains daily will help you achieve the RDA for fiber (about 25 grams per day for women and 35 grams per day for men). Choose from a wide variety of grains, including quinoa, oatmeal, whole wheat pasta, flax seeds and bran cereal.

EYEFOODS
Barley, bran cereal, brown rice, buckwheat, bulgur, farro, flax seeds, oats, quinoa, wheat berries, whole wheat pasta, other whole grains

EYE NUTRIENTS
Fiber, vitamin E, zinc

WEEKLY TARGET
- $1/2$ cup (125 mL) cooked grains, four times a week; eat a variety of whole grains

---

DID YOU KNOW?

Heart-Healthy Is Eye-Healthy

The *British Journal of Ophthalmology* published a study in 2008 showing that people with AMD have a higher risk of developing cardiovascular disease. Because AMD and cardiovascular disease share many common risk factors, a heart-friendly diet is an eye-friendly diet, and increasing your fiber intake will contribute to healthy blood vessels and eyes.

BE AWARE

- Not all whole grains have a low glycemic index. For example, whole wheat bread and white bread have a similar glycemic index. Good whole-grain choices include quinoa, buckwheat and steel-cut oats.
- Watch your serving size. Even though they are loaded with health benefits, whole grains contain a similar amount of calories to refined grains.
- When purchasing breakfast cereals, look for products that are low in sugar and that contain 100% whole grains. Be aware of marketing schemes and misleading nutritional claims on the packaging. The best choices are products that have a fiber content of at least 3 grams per 100 calories and a sugar content no higher than 10 grams per 100 calories.

Gluten-Free Diets

Whether you suffer from celiac disease or are sensitive to gluten, if you are following a gluten-free diet, these lists will help you choose appropriate whole grains:

Grains That Contain Gluten

• Barley	• Farro	• Semolina	• Wheat
• Bulgur	• Kamut	• Spelt	• Wheat berries
• Durum wheat	• Rye	• Triticale	

Gluten-Free Grains

• Amaranth	• Corn	• Oats (if packaged without cross-contamination)	• Quinoa
• Buckwheat	• Millet		• Rice

Barley

Barley is an ancient grain that is commonly used in soups. It has a nutty flavor and chewy texture and can be enjoyed in place of pasta or rice in salads or as a base for stir-fries. Barley comes in hulled, pearl and pot varieties. Hulled barley remains a whole grain, as the outer husk — which is not digestible by humans — is the only part removed; the bran and germ remain. Hulled barley takes longer to cook than pot or pearl barley, but offers more nutrition.

Because some of the outer bran layer is removed from pearl and pot barley (more from pearl than from pot), they are technically not whole grains; however, they are still more nutritious than other refined grains and are higher in fiber.

Brown Rice

The whole-grain version of rice packs more of a nutritional punch than its refined white counterpart, containing more vitamins, minerals and fiber. Brown rice is available in short-, medium- and long-grain varieties.

Buckwheat

Despite its name, buckwheat is actually not a wheat and does not contain gluten. It is a healthy whole grain that can be used in place of pasta and rice. Raw buckwheat has a crunchy texture and a nutty flavor. When cooked, buckwheat has a similar texture to rice. Soba noodles, popular in Japanese cuisine, are made from buckwheat flour. Buckwheat flour can also be used to make pancakes and crêpes.

See page 178 for simple cooking instructions for a variety of whole grains.

Bulgur

Made from parboiled wheat groats, bulgur cooks in no time, making it a quick weeknight option.

Farro

This ancient wheat strain has a wonderful chewy texture and is a great swap for barley in recipes. It comes in whole-grain, semi-pearled and pearled varieties. Make sure to choose whole-grain for the best nutrition, even though it has a longer cooking time.

Flax Seeds

Flax seeds have significant amounts of the omega-3 fatty acid ALA, fiber, vitamin E and zinc. Keep in mind that flax seeds should be consumed in addition to fish, not as a substitute for it. Our bodies do convert ALA to DHA and EPA (the omega-3 fatty acids that are abundant in fish and are most used by our bodies), but not very efficiently.

DID YOU KNOW?

Grinding Flax Seeds

Grind your flax seeds using a coffee or spice grinder. Our bodies cannot break down the outer coating of the whole seed, so the seed exits our body intact and we do not absorb any nutrients. Coarsely ground flax is stable at room temperature and will remain fresh for up to 10 months.

Oats

Oats have the highest proportion of soluble fiber of all grains. If purchasing prepared oatmeal, choose unsweetened plain oatmeal and add a small amount of honey or maple syrup to sweeten it. Or make your own oatmeal from quick-cooking rolled oats or steel-cut oats.

Quinoa

This nutty-tasting grain is a complete protein, making it a great choice for meatless diets. Along with bulgur and wheat berries, quinoa is becoming much easier to find in supermarkets these days. It is easy to prepare and will add variety to your diet.

Wheat Berries

Containing all three parts of the grain — the germ, the bran and the endosperm — wheat berries are unrefined and high in fiber. They take 45 to 60 minutes to cook, and their chewy texture makes them a great addition to soups, stews and salads.

Beans and Lentils

Beans and lentils are a great source of fiber and protein and contain a minimal amount of fat, so they are an integral part of an eye-healthy, heart-healthy diet. Romano beans and black beans are the top eyefoods in this category because they are very rich in fiber and contain significant amounts of zinc. Soybeans (edamame) also score well as an eyefood thanks to their high content of the omega-3 fatty acid ALA.

The easiest way to include beans and lentils in your diet is to buy them canned. However, canned beans and lentils tend to have a high sodium content, so rinse them thoroughly. Alternatively, you can buy dried beans and lentils, soak them as necessary and cook them yourself.

Edamame are available in the pod or shelled, and can be found in the freezer section of your grocery store.

EYEFOODS

Black beans, black lentils, brown lentils, cannellini (white kidney) beans, chickpeas, green lentils, red kidney beans, red lentils, Romano beans, soybeans (edamame)

TOP EYEFOODS

Romano beans, black beans, soybeans (edamame)

EYE NUTRIENTS

Fiber, omega-3 fatty acids (ALA), zinc

WEEKLY TARGET

- $1/2$ cup (125 mL) cooked beans or lentils, four times a week

DID YOU KNOW?

Bean Cuisine

Many different cultures use beans and lentils in their cuisine. East Indian cuisine features lentils, Mediterranean cuisine includes Romano and cannellini (white kidney) beans, Mexican cuisine relies on red kidney and black beans, and Asian cuisine makes good use of soybeans. Even the typical North American diet includes beans, mainly the navy beans found in baked beans.

Meal and Snack Ideas

- Make a colorful bean salad with canned beans, orange bell peppers, sun-dried tomatoes and green onions.
- Enjoy hummus (chickpea spread) as a sandwich spread or dip.
- Serve edamame in the pod as an appetizer. Sprinkle them with salt and eat them with your fingers. Avoid eating the pod, as it is very tough; just run the pod through your teeth to scrape out the seeds.
- For a crunchy snack, toss cooked cannellini (white kidney) beans or chickpeas with olive oil and your favorite mix of spices. (Try ground cumin, curry powder and ground coriander.) Roast in a 400°F (200°C) oven for 40 minutes.

Eyefoods Tips: Beans and Lentils

- Rinse canned beans well in a colander under running water to get rid of excess sodium.
- Add cooked beans to soups, stews and sautés.
- Serve cooked green lentils instead of rice as a side dish for fish.
- Add shelled edamame to stir-fries, soups and salads.
- Drink plenty of water to avoid the gassy effects of eating beans.

Healthy Fats

Olive oil and flaxseed oil are monounsaturated fats that contain vitamin E and the omega-3 fatty acid ALA. Other healthy oils include walnut oil, grapeseed oil and avocado oil. Walnut oil is a nice treat in a delicate salad. Grapeseed and avocado oils have a high smoke point, making them good choices for a stir-fry.

EYEFOODS
Avocado oil, flaxseed oil, grapeseed oil, olive oil, walnut oil

TOP EYEFOOD
Olive oil

EYE NUTRIENTS
Omega-3 fatty acids (ALA), vitamin E

DAILY TARGET
- 1 to 2 tablespoons (15 to 30 mL) per day

Olive Oil

Olive oil is derived from the fat of olives and is a staple in the Mediterranean diet. It is sold in different grades: extra virgin, virgin, regular and light. Virgin and extra virgin olive oil are not treated with chemicals or altered by heat; the olives are simply pressed to extract the oil. While both oils are unrefined, extra virgin oil must pass stricter quality control tests. It is more flavorful but also more expensive. It has a lower smoke point and degrades when heated above 375°F (190°C). For the full benefit of its intense flavor and its nutrients, extra virgin olive oil is best enjoyed on salads or drizzled on dishes after cooking.

Regular and light olive oil are refined products and therefore have fewer nutrients than the unrefined oils. They are less expensive, have a milder flavor and have a higher smoke point, which makes them better suited to higher-heat cooking methods such as stir-frying, searing or grilling.

> ### Eyefoods Tips: Healthy Fats
>
> - Use olive oil instead of butter as often as you can.
> - Choose extra virgin olive oil as much as possible. It comes from the first press and has the best flavor and the most health benefits.
> - Once it's opened, store flaxseed oil in the refrigerator and use it up within 6 weeks.

Pro Tip

Remember that fat from any source is calorie-dense. To avoid an expanding waistline, eat a minimal amount.

Chapter 6

Lifestyle and General Health

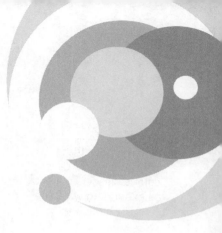

Patients ask me every day how they can protect their vision. This chapter will explain how your lifestyle decisions can benefit your eyes and your everyday life.

We all know that proper nutrition is essential to our well-being. In addition to promoting long-term overall health, good eating habits will nourish your eyes. But other parts of your lifestyle also directly affect the health of your eyes. For instance, smoking increases the risk for age-related macular degeneration (AMD), and regular exercise can help prevent certain eye diseases.

My lifestyle recommendations for preventing eye disease will also promote long-term general health. The benefits of a healthy lifestyle are numerous. You will notice that you have the energy and vitality you need to lead a happy and fulfilling life.

Eating eyefoods will lead you down the path to better eye health, but an overall healthy lifestyle will have an even greater impact on the prevention of eye disease. The eye-friendly lifestyle recommendations in this chapter will help you improve your eye health and general well-being.

Ultraviolet and Blue Light Exposure

The sun and certain types of lamps, such as those used in tanning beds, emit ultraviolet (UV) radiation. Researchers have found that overexposure to UV light may cause cataracts, AMD, skin cancer, sunburns and premature aging of the skin. The U.S. Food and Drug Administration (FDA) recommends wearing sunglasses, using sunscreen to protect against the harmful effects of UV light and avoiding overexposure to UV light and tanning beds. Health Canada says "There is no such thing as a safe tan" and, in an article titled "It's Your Health: Tanning Lamps," available online, has published advice on making informed decisions when using a tanning bed.

Blue light (short-wavelength visible light) causes oxidative stress to the retina. This affects people with less of the macular pigments lutein and zeaxanthin. People with light-colored irises, people with AMD and people with a genetic predisposition to AMD are more susceptible to the harmful effects of blue light.

Pro Tip

Overexposure to UV light may cause skin cancer, sunburn and premature aging of the skin.

Childhood UV Light Exposure

Babies, children and young adults have more transparent lenses in their eyes and more sensitive skin. As a result, they are at a greater risk of experiencing the adverse effects of overexposure to UV light — though those effects may not show up until later in life. By 18 years of age, the average person has received 80% of their life's UV exposure. That's why it is critical to effectively protect our children's eyes from the sun, beginning at birth and continuing throughout their childhood.

Choosing Sunglasses

When it comes to choosing sunglasses, the options are endless, which can be confusing without some important background information. Not all lenses are equal in terms of UV and blue light protection. The optical quality of the lens, the level of protection and the longevity of such protection vary greatly. Here are a few helpful tips:

- **Visible light and UV light:** The light spectrum is categorized by wavelength. If the light is in the visible spectrum, the wavelengths will determine its color. If it is in the UV range, the wavelengths determine its UV category (A, B or C).
- **Blue wavelength light:** Blue wavelength light can damage the retina, leading to AMD and blurring of vision.
- **Types of glare:** Direct glare is the bright light that comes from the sun above and its reflection below. Reflected glare is produced by flat, smooth and shiny surfaces, like a car windshield, the surface of a lake or puddles on the road. Bounce-back glare reaches you from the side and from behind.

The difference between a high-quality and a low-quality pair of sunglasses is determined by their UV protection and by how well they filter blue light. The gold standard in sunglasses for UV protection has until recently been UV 400, which protects against UV categories A, B and C. We now know that visible blue light also has damaging effects on the eyes, so optimal sun protection includes a selective blue filter. The once-popular "Blue Blocker" lens blocked all blue light rays, but it also changed the quality of the colors seen through the glasses. Newer lenses allow you to see colors normally while still absorbing the damaging energy of blue light.

Lens Features

- The color, or tint, of a sunglasses lens does not affect the quality of its UV and blue light protection. In fact, you can get a clear UV 400 coating on your lenses. Cheaply made UV 400 sunglasses have a spray-on coating that will wear off with cleaning, giving you a false sense of security, and not all brands of lenses have blue light filters. A high-quality pair of sunglasses will filter blue light as well as UV light.

- A mirror on the front of your lenses will reflect most of the direct glare, essentially "squinting" so you don't have to.

- A polarized filter eliminates reflected glare from the road, water, windshields and other flat, shiny surfaces. With polarized lenses, you can see below the water's surface, so they are great for fishing.

- A back surface antireflective coating prevents light from bouncing off the back of the lens and into your eyes. This feature reduces glare.

- A photochromic lens adjusts to lighting conditions, getting darker as the light gets brighter. It is activated by UV rays, so it will not get as dark when you are inside a car as it does when you are outside.

- Excellent-quality plastic lenses will be impact-resistant, lightweight and treated with an anti-scratch coating. They will have high-quality optics, giving you sharper vision.

- Glass lenses are heavier and more resistant to scratching, and provide crisp optics. Because they are not impact-resistant and may shatter, they are not well-suited to sports use.

- You can choose the color of the tint of your sunglasses depending on your visual needs, how you intend to use your sunglasses and your personal preference. Brown tints increase contrast; gray tints do not alter color perception.

Pro Tip

Specialized tints are available for different sports and activities. You can get lenses that maximize your vision for tennis, golf, hunting and fishing, to name a few.

Frames

- When choosing the frame for your sunglasses, the most important thing to consider is fit. The frame should fit close to your eyes and face to reduce the entry of bounce-back glare, and it must be big enough to provide appropriate coverage and protection for your eyes.

- Most quality sunglasses are available with your prescription, so you don't have to put up with wearing one pair of glasses on top of another.

- Clip-on sunglasses are available for most prescription glasses. Although these are an acceptable compromise, they add to the weight of your glasses, causing them to slip down your nose. There will also be internal reflection between the two sets of lenses, which decreases the quality of your vision. With frequent use, the clip may cause paint to chip off your frame.

- If you choose a clip-on or a photochromic lens, you should be aware that light will still reach your eyes from around the frame. This is because regular eyeglasses are usually smaller and flatter than sunglasses, and do not fit as close to your face.

Computer and Device Use

Do you come home from work or school feeling like your eyes have been glued to the computer — literally? Are you having a hard time falling asleep after late-night emails or Candy Crush? These technology tips will help improve your visual comfort and performance at home, work and play.

Remember to Blink!

Our blink rate decreases from approximately 17 times per minute to 10 times per minute when we are using electronic devices or really concentrating on a specific activity. A decreased blink rate can result in dryness, discomfort and even blurry or distorted vision. Make sure you are fully closing your eyes while blinking — research shows that partial blinking at a faster rate is the same as barely blinking at all!

20/20/20 Rule

Every 20 minutes, focus on an object at least 20 feet away for 20 seconds. Taking regular breaks from our electronic devices allows our eyes to relax and reduces strain throughout the day. You can set an alarm to help you remember to take these regular "daydream breaks." There are even computer programs, such as Google's eyeCare, available to give you scheduled reminders.

Invest in Your Vision

When updating your glasses, invest in a good antireflective coating and blue light filter. This filter absorbs some of the high-energy blue light being emitted from our electronic devices and decreases the amount that is transmitted into our eyes. As a result, your eyes will feel less strain and fatigue throughout the day and night.

Optimize Your Workspace to Maximize Your Vision

- Keep your computer monitor or laptop at arm's length and 15 to 20 degrees below eye level.
- Match the brightness and contrast of your screen to your surroundings.
- Minimize sources of glare on your screen. Position your monitor or laptop so that natural or diffuse lighting is on either side of your workstation. Light should not be directed in front of or behind your screen.
- Increase clarity by removing all dirt and dust from electronic screens.

Avoid Blue Light Before Bed

At night, the blue light emitted by our devices can disrupt our circadian rhythm and melatonin production, making it harder to fall asleep. The best way to avoid sleep disruption is to put down your devices and say good night to technology at least 2 hours before bedtime.

> ### DID YOU KNOW?
>
> **There's an App for That**
>
> For those who aren't able to kick the late-night tech habit, there are smartphone and tablet apps that modify brightness settings and filter the amount of blue light being emitted as day progresses into night.

FAQ

Q. How can I minimize the effects of blue light?

A. We can decrease our exposure to blue light by restricting technology use and using applications that decrease the amount of blue light emitted by our smartphones and computers. It's also important to have a blue light filter on both your prescription glasses and sunglasses.

Another way to protect the macula from these high-energy rays is to increase your intake of lutein and zeaxanthin. These carotenoids are concentrated in the macula, where they act as blue light filters. Our bodies do not make lutein or zeaxanthin, so it is important to obtain these pigments through diet or supplements. Kale is the top food choice for blue light protection — 1 cup (250 mL) contains 10 milligrams of lutein. Watercress, pea shoots and Chinese broccoli are also good, often-overlooked, leafy greens choices.

I recommend making leafy greens a daily addition to your diet by adding them to salads, soups or smoothies. Eating orange bell peppers (both raw and cooked) and eggs four times per week will also help increase the concentration of lutein and zeaxanthin in your body and maculae.

Smoking

The dangerous effects of smoking have long been proven. Most people are well aware that smoking greatly increases the risk of cancer and heart disease, but other parts of the body are affected as well. Studies show that smoking is the most important modifiable risk factor in AMD. Compared to people who have never smoked, current smokers are 45% more likely to develop early AMD or have their AMD progress over a period of 15 years. For information on quitting smoking, visit www.smokefree.gov or breakitoff.ca.

Body Mass Index and Waist Circumference

The United States Department of Agriculture (USDA) and Health Canada recommend maintaining a healthy body weight to help prevent chronic disease and improve your general health. The World Health Organization (WHO), USDA and Health Canada recognize body mass index (BMI) and waist circumference as the two measurements used by professionals to help determine a person's risk for developing diseases associated with being overweight. (Note that these tools do not apply to children under the age of 18 or to pregnant or lactating women.)

- **BMI:** BMI is a ratio of weight to height. You can calculate your BMI by consulting an online BMI table or by using the formula BMI = weight (kg)/height (m)^2. A normal BMI is between 18.5 and 24.9. A BMI over 25 is in the overweight category, and a BMI over 30 is in the obese category. People in the overweight or obese categories have a higher risk of developing health problems.

- **Waist circumference:** Waist circumference is an indicator of abdominal obesity. Many health professionals recognize that people with an apple-shaped body — men with a waist circumference greater than 40 inches (100 cm) and women with a waist circumference greater than 35 inches (87.5 cm) — have an increased risk of developing certain chronic health conditions.

Mindful Eating

The concept of mindful eating involves being present in the moment while you are eating, as well as when you are shopping for and preparing your food. Practicing mindful eating can help you lose weight. Pay attention to the color, texture, aroma and taste of your food. Eat slowly, taking small bites and chewing thoroughly. If you are eating with friends or family, try to devote your first few bites to being mindful before you start chatting. If you are eating alone, shun the TV or devices and focus on your food.

Physical Activity

We all know the long-term health benefits of exercise, but making physical activity a regular part of your life will also help you feel younger, stronger and more energetic right now. Physical activity stimulates blood circulation, nourishing and detoxifying your cells. It benefits your heart and arteries, and therefore your eyes and vision. Increased physical activity can decrease the risk of cardiovascular disease and stroke. Other health benefits include weight control, stronger muscles and bones, reduced stress and increased energy and vitality.

I recommend regular physical activity as part of an eye-friendly lifestyle. Exercise daily. Go for a walk or enjoy the scenery on a bike ride. Aim for the following targets:

- **Adults:** 30 to 60 minutes of physical activity per day
- **Children and youth:** 90 minutes of physical activity per day

If you have any health concerns, consult your physician before starting any new exercise program.

Pro Tip

Scientists believe that exercising at least three times a week can slow the progression of AMD.

Research Spotlight

Cardiovascular Disease and AMD

Current scientific studies show a relationship between AMD and cardiovascular disease; independently, long-standing research on each of these diseases demonstrates similar findings. They share many of the same risk factors, including age, smoking, antioxidant levels, physical activity, BMI and waist circumference.

In 2006, scientists found that patients with late AMD had a 30.9% increased risk of coronary heart disease over 10 years, while patients with no signs of AMD had only a 10% increased risk of coronary heart disease over the same period. Patients with late AMD also had a higher incidence of stroke than patients without any signs of AMD. Another study found that people with AMD between the ages of 49 and 75 had a greater long-term risk of having serious complications related to cardiovascular disease and stroke.

Many commonalities exist between eye-friendly and heart-friendly lifestyles, including good nutrition, physical activity and not smoking.

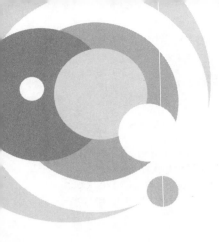

Chapter 7

Following the Eyefoods Plan

In the previous chapters, I discussed the food and lifestyle choices that can reduce your risk of developing age-related macular degeneration (AMD), cataracts, dry eye syndrome and eyelid disorders. I identified the nutrients that offer the greatest protection against eye disease, and I introduced eyefoods, the foods that are richest in these nutrients. In this chapter, I offer the Eyefoods Plan, a simple way to integrate eyefoods into your life. Following the Eyefoods Plan will help you prevent eye disease and maintain a strong, healthy body, while also reducing your risk of developing other chronic diseases.

The Eyefoods Plan outlines weekly targets for eyefoods. It offers simple ways to identify serving sizes and track your weekly eyefood consumption. It also provides guidelines on other lifestyle factors that are important to eye health, including eye supplements, sun protection, smoking, exercise and weight management.

The Eyefoods Plan is meant to be a complement to a healthy diet and lifestyle. You will need to consume more food on a weekly basis than what is recommended in the Eyefoods Plan. For the remainder of your food intake, follow the guidelines set by the "Dietary Guidelines for Americans" or "Eating Well with Canada's Food Guide."

> The Eyefoods Plan is based on scientific research on nutrition and eye health. It gives you an easy way to incorporate eyefoods and eye-healthy lifestyle choices into your life.

Weekly Targets

To determine the recommended intake of each of the eye nutrients for the Eyefoods Plan, Dr. Pelletier and I paid particular attention to the Age-Related Eye Disease Study (AREDS) and the dietary reference intakes recommended by the United States Department of Agriculture (USDA) and Health Canada. We also studied the nutrient values of hundreds of whole foods and considered how a reasonable diet could include these nutrients.

The Eyefoods Nutrition Plan (page 115) meets all of the weekly targets listed on page 113 except zinc. In addition to following the Eyefoods Nutrition Plan, you will need to include whole grains and dairy or dairy alternative food choices from USDA's My Plate or Canada's Food Guide in your diet. These additional foods will help you achieve the zinc target.

> ### • CAUTION •
>
> The Eyefoods Plan is not meant to replace an eye vitamin for people who are at high risk for eye disease or who already have diagnosed eye disease. Rather, this plan is a recommended course of action for leading a lifestyle that promotes eye health and overall physical well-being.

Finding Trustworthy Health Resources

There is a seemingly endless selection of health resources available to us today, particularly in the media and on the web. The diverse recommendations and reports can cause confusion. Sometimes, health topics reported in the media can conflict with recommendations you have received from your health care provider. Be aware that not all published information on health is trustworthy. Scientific research should be the foundation of any health-related publication or recommendation. It is important to seek out reliable sources that back up their findings with accurate scientific research.

Reliable information can be found in many publications from government agencies, health care foundations and universities. When Dr. Pelletier and I developed the Eyefoods Plan, we consulted dietary and lifestyle guidelines and recommendations from the United States Department of Agriculture (USDA), the American Heart Association, the American Cancer Society, Health Canada, the Heart and Stroke Foundation and the Canadian Cancer Society, as well as current scientific studies in the field of nutrition and eye health. A registered dietitian reviewed and verified the information in the Eyefoods Plan.

Eyefoods Target Nutrients

Scientific studies show that the following nutrients may help prevent eye disease. The Eyefoods Nutrition Plan includes foods that provide all of these nutrients.

Nutrient	Eyefoods Daily Target	Eyefoods Weekly Target
Beta-carotene	10 mg	70 mg
Lutein and zeaxanthin	10 mg	70 mg
Vitamin C	350 mg	2,450 mg
Vitamin E	15 mg	105 mg
Zinc	10 mg	70 mg
Fiber	30 g	210 g
Omega-3 fatty acids from fish (DHA/EPA)	0.85 g	5.95 g
Omega-3 fatty acids from plants (ALA)	1.6 g	11.2 g

Serving Sizes

Most nutrition and diet plans offer serving size suggestions that can be confusing. When you're following a nutrition plan, proper serving sizes are important to ensure that you receive enough of the recommended nutrients from your food. The Eyefoods Plan recommends serving sizes that allow you to obtain optimal health benefits from each food while maintaining appropriate portion control.

With our busy lifestyles, we don't usually have time to weigh or measure each food we eat to determine the proper serving size. The chart below offers simple guidelines you can use to quickly determine the serving size of certain foods.

Serving Sizes

Scientific studies show that the following nutrients may help prevent eye disease. The Eyefoods Nutrition Plan includes foods that provide all of these nutrients.

Food	Eyefoods Serving Size	Handy Guideline
Raw leafy green vegetables	1 cup (250 mL)	1 large handful
Other vegetables	½ cup (125 mL)	Size of a small lemon
Fruit	½ cup (125 mL) chopped fruit, 1 medium fruit or 4 dried apricots	Size of a small lemon (for the chopped fruit)
Cold-water fish and lean protein	3½ oz (100 g) cooked	Size of a deck of cards
Nuts	½ oz (16 g)	1 small handful
Whole grains	½ cup (125 mL) cooked grains or 1 thin slice of bread	Size of a small lemon (for the cooked grains)
Oils	1 tbsp (15 mL)	

The Eyefoods Nutrition Plan

This plan outlines how much of each eyefood you should eat on a weekly or daily basis to reach your eye nutrient targets. Following the nutrition plan will ensure that you are nourishing your eyes with high amounts of beta-carotene, lutein and zeaxanthin, omega-3 fatty acids, vitamin C, vitamin E and zinc.

Category	Foods	Eyefoods Target
Cooked leafy green vegetables	Kale, spinach, dandelion greens, Swiss chard, other leafy greens	$\frac{1}{2}$ cup (125 mL), twice a week
Raw leafy green vegetables	Kale, spinach, radicchio, romaine, other dark green lettuces	1 cup (250 mL), seven times a week; choose kale and spinach often
Cold-water fish	Salmon, sardines, tuna, mackerel, rainbow trout	$3\frac{1}{2}$ oz (100 g) cooked, four times a week: two servings of salmon and two of other cold-water fish
Cooked orange vegetables	Sweet potatoes, butternut squash, carrots, pumpkin	$\frac{1}{2}$ cup (125 mL), three times a week
Raw carrots	Carrot sticks, shredded carrot, carrot juice	$\frac{1}{2}$ cup (125 mL), three times a week
Orange bell peppers	Orange bell peppers	$\frac{1}{2}$ pepper, four times a week (2 servings raw, 2 servings cooked)
Green vegetables	Broccoli (especially raw broccoli), Brussels sprouts, green peas	$\frac{1}{2}$ cup (125 mL), seven times a week
Eggs	Eggs high in omega-3 fatty acids	2 eggs, twice a week (a total of 4 eggs a week)
Fruit	Kiwifruit, cantaloupe, avocado, apricots (dried and fresh), other fruits	3 servings per day
Fruit juice	Orange juice, apple juice, pineapple juice, Concord grape juice, pomegranate juice, lemon juice	1 cup (250 mL) unsweetened fruit juice per day; add 2 tbsp (30 mL) lemon juice to water or tea each day
Lean protein	Turkey breast, lean cuts of beef	$3\frac{1}{2}$ oz (100 g) cooked turkey breast, four times a week; $3\frac{1}{2}$ oz (100 g) cooked lean beef, twice a week
Nuts and seeds	Eyefoods Nut Mix (page 222), flax seeds, wheat germ	1 small handful of Eyefoods Nut Mix per day
Whole grains	Oatmeal, quinoa, spelt, whole-grain bread, whole-grain pasta, other whole grains	$\frac{1}{2}$ cup (125 mL) cooked, five times a week
Beans and lentils	Romano beans, black beans, soybeans (edamame), cannellini (white kidney) beans, chickpeas, lentils, red kidney beans	$\frac{1}{2}$ cup (125 mL) cooked, four times a week
Oils	Olive oil, walnut oil, grapeseed oil, avocado oil	1–2 tbsp (15–30 mL) per day

The Eyefoods Lifestyle Plan

- Follow the Eyefoods Nutrition Plan above.

- Wear good-quality sunglasses. See your eye care professional for advice on the best type of sunglasses for you.

- Take control of your health. Seek out the services of an eye care professional, a family physician and any other necessary health care providers. Visit them regularly and have them work as a team for you.

- Get moving. Exercise daily. Go for a walk or a bike ride, dance with your family and learn a new sport or activity. It will bring balance to your life and make you smile more!

- Quit smoking. Visit www.smokefree.gov or breakitoff.ca, or consult your family physician for help.

- Take an eye vitamin. If you are at risk for developing eye disease, have eye disease or cannot reach the eyefoods targets through your diet, take an eye vitamin. Consult your eye care provider about the best supplement for you.

- Maintain a healthy weight. If you follow the Eyefoods Plan, you will be on your way to achieving this goal.

Plant a Garden to Keep Your Eyes and Body Healthy

A backyard garden is a great way to complement a healthy lifestyle. We've known for years that including a variety of fruits and vegetables in our diet helps keep our bodies healthy and prevent chronic disease. In more recent years, the concern over environmental toxins has caused a rapid increase in the number of people who are growing their own produce in their backyard. Fruits and vegetables contain their highest amount of nutrients when they are first harvested, so that's the best time to eat them!

Here are some tips to help you plant fruits and vegetables that will provide an array of disease-fighting nutrients:

- Create a garden with a variety of colors.
- Enjoy your fruits and vegetables as soon as possible after picking them, when they are at their most nutritious.
- Plant early and late varieties of vegetables to ensure that you have options throughout the growing season.
- Include various herbs, such as parsley, basil, mint, thyme, sage, oregano and cilantro, in your garden. Herbs have disease-fighting properties and are a great way to add healthy flavor to salads and other fresh vegetable dishes.

If You Follow a Paleo Diet

The paleo diet, developed in 2002 by Dr. Loren Cordain, is based on the theory that the optimal diet for humans is one to which we are genetically adapted. Human DNA has not changed much in the past 40,000 years, yet our diet has changed dramatically with industrialization and the agricultural revolution. The paleo diet closely follows the hunter-gatherer diet of our ancestors from the Paleolithic era. Here are the foods you can eat on the paleo diet:

- Lean meats (preferably from grass-fed animals) or fish at every meal
- Unlimited fruits and non-starchy vegetables
- Nuts and seeds in moderation

Processed foods and foods that are high in sugar are not allowed on a strict paleo diet. These include:

- Cereals and grains (pasta, crackers, rice, barley, oatmeal)
- Legumes (peanuts, peas, lentils)
- Starchy vegetables (potatoes and sweet potatoes)
- Dairy products
- Processed meats (bacon, hot dogs, deli meats)
- Soft drinks, sweets

Pro Tip

Grass-fed meat tends to be leaner than grain-fed and has higher amounts of omega-3 fatty acids.

The paleo diet includes a relatively high amount of animal protein compared to a typical North American diet. However, by choosing fish and lean meats such as turkey breast, chicken breast and grass-fed beef tenderloin, and avoiding processed meats, you will be consuming only a moderate amount of fat. In addition, if you choose grass-fed meat and consume a high amount of fish, you will have a lower omega-6:omega-3 ratio, which helps combat inflammation.

People following a paleo diet tend to have a large intake of fiber, as they consume healthy carbohydrates in the form of fruits and vegetables. Foods restricted on the paleo diet are processed and refined carbohydrates, which tend to have a high glycemic index and have been shown to increase the risk for obesity and cardiovascular disease.

Eye-Healthy Foods on a Paleo Diet

If you follow a paleo diet, the following tips will ensure that you receive adequate amounts of the nutrients important for ocular health and function, such as lutein, zeaxanthin, vitamin C, vitamin E, zinc, DHA and EPA:

> Both paleo and plant-based diets have the potential to include a significant amount of fruits and vegetables, which are rich in phytochemicals, vitamins, minerals and antioxidants.

- Choose the following vegetables: leafy greens, orange bell peppers, broccoli, Brussels sprouts.
- Choose the following fruits: kiwifruit, cantaloupe, avocado, berries, citrus fruits.
- Eat four eggs per week.
- Consume fish, especially salmon, sardines, light tuna, mackerel and rainbow trout, four times a week.
- Eat a handful of nuts every day. Good nut choices include almonds, walnuts, cashews and pistachios.

What's Missing?

Whole grains, beans and lentils are eyefoods that aren't part of the paleo diet. One of the main reasons that these foods are important for eye health is that they tend to have a high fiber content. People who are following the paleo diet properly should have a high fiber intake thanks to eating a lot of fruits and vegetables, so omitting whole grains, beans and lentils shouldn't be an issue.

If You Follow a Plant-Based Diet

Population surveys done between 2008 and 2013 found that between 3% and 13% of North Americans follow a vegetarian or vegan diet for social, cultural or health reasons. Vegetarians and vegans often maintain their diet for a lifetime, unlike other diet trends that people may follow for only a short period.

A vegan or vegetarian diet typically includes a lot of fruits and vegetables, which provide high amounts of antioxidants and carotenoids. However, plant-based diets that eliminate all meat, fish and dairy may be lacking in the important ocular nutrients zinc, vitamin E and the omega-3 fatty acids DHA and EPA.

People who don't eat fish will likely have a low intake of DHA and EPA. To compensate, eat plant sources of omega-3s (ALA) or take a vegan omega-3 supplement. Foods high in ALA include flax seeds, walnuts, avocados, soy products and chia seeds. Our bodies can convert ALA into DHA and EPA; however, this conversion is not very efficient, so you may be receiving inadequate amounts of DHA and EPA even when consuming ALA-rich foods. For this reason, I often recommend that my patients who follow a vegan diet take a high-quality vegan omega-3 supplement.

Another eye-healthy food that may be missing in a plant-based diet is eggs, which contain high amounts of lutein, vitamin E, zinc and DHA (in omega-3 eggs). Eggs are an important source of lutein, as the lutein from eggs is very bioavailable. The fat in eggs, and the lack of chlorophyll, allows the lutein to be absorbed well by our bodies. To compensate for not eating eggs, it is important to eat more leafy greens and green vegetables. I recommend eating at least a handful of leafy green vegetables a day, along with a healthy fat (such as extra virgin olive oil) to aid in the absorption of lutein.

Zinc and vitamin E intake may also be low in vegan diets, as meat, fish and eggs are good sources of these nutrients. Replace the zinc by consuming lots of beans, lentils and whole grains. To increase your intake of vitamin E, eat almonds, sunflower seeds, leafy greens, orange bell peppers, wheat germ and olive oil.

Pro Tip

Seaweed, such as the nori found in sushi rolls, and micro-algae are non-fish food sources of DHA.

Research Spotlight
Plant-Based Diets and Lower Mortality Rates

Research that supports plant-based diets includes the 20-year China–Cornell–Oxford Project. This study looked at mortality rates from cancer and other chronic diseases in 65 counties in China, and concluded that the counties with a higher consumption of animal-based foods had higher death rates from chronic diseases than counties that favored plant-based diets.

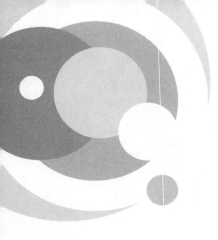

Chapter 8

Integrating Eyefoods into Your Diet

Eyefood Focus

Adding a handful of leafy greens, such as kale or spinach, to your daily diet is a simple habit that will greatly increase the amount of lutein you consume.

You have taken the first step toward taking better care of your eyes by learning about eye anatomy, common eye diseases and the nutrients, foods and lifestyle habits that may help decrease the risk for chronic eye diseases such as age-related macular degeneration, cataracts and dry eye syndrome. You may already have started making better everyday choices that will lead to a lifetime of healthier eyes. Now it's time to really start putting your acquired knowledge to practical use.

A good way to start incorporating eyefoods into your diet is to devote a meal a day to your eye health. This chapter offers sample weekly meal plans, along with grocery shopping lists and lists of "must have" foods for your pantry and freezer, to help you do just that. The meal plans incorporate recipes from Part 3: Recipes for Healthy Eyes — delicious, easy dishes that are chock-full of eyefoods.

Four Simple Eyefood Tips

If you want to start incorporating eyefoods into your diet, but feel overwhelmed by the Eyefoods Plan, these four simple tips will help you enjoy the most important eye-healthy foods:

- Eat a handful of leafy green vegetables per day. Try kale, spinach, dandelion greens, collard greens, romaine lettuce and radicchio, both raw and cooked.
- Eat two orange bell peppers per week, both raw and cooked.
- Eat cold-water fish two to four times per week. Salmon, rainbow trout, sardines, light tuna and mackerel are all good choices.
- Eat four eggs per week — the yolk is full of good stuff!

Track It!

To ensure that you are receiving enough eye-healthy nutrients to nourish your eyes and help prevent eye disease, you need to know how much of each eyefood to consume, then keep track of your intake of these foods. Use the table below to monitor the type and amount of eyefoods you are consuming.

Food	Eat This Many Servings Weekly
Cooked leafy greens	◯ ◯
Raw leafy greens	◯ ◯ ◯ ◯ ◯ ◯ ◯
Cold-water fish	◯ ◯ ◯ ◯
Cooked orange vegetables	◯ ◯ ◯
Raw carrots	◯ ◯ ◯
Orange bell peppers	◯ ◯ ◯ ◯
Green vegetables	◯ ◯ ◯ ◯ ◯ ◯ ◯
Eggs	◯ ◯ ◯ ◯
Fruit	◯ ◯
Fruit juice	◯ ◯ ◯ ◯ ◯ ◯ ◯
Lean protein	◯ ◯ ◯ ◯ ◯ ◯
Nuts and seeds	◯ ◯ ◯ ◯ ◯ ◯ ◯
Whole grains	◯ ◯ ◯ ◯ ◯
Beans and lentils	◯ ◯ ◯ ◯
Olive oil	◯ ◯ ◯ ◯ ◯ ◯ ◯ ◯ ◯ ◯ ◯ ◯ ◯ ◯

A Meal a Day for Healthy Eyes

Once you feel comfortable with these weekly meal plans, you can start to create your own plans by choosing one meal per day and preparing one or two eyefood recipes for that meal. A time-saving tip is to prepare enough of each recipe so that you have leftovers for the next day. This will also help to increase your intake of eyefoods.

Sample Weekly Meal Plans

It's easy to devote a meal a day to healthy eyes. These weekly plans show you how.

Week 1	
MONDAY LUNCH	Turkey and Swiss sandwich: grilled turkey slices on whole-grain bread, with mustard, romaine lettuce, sun-dried tomatoes and Swiss cheese Orange bell pepper slices with Hummus (page 226) Fresh-squeezed orange juice with a splash of lemon juice
TUESDAY DINNER	Grilled salmon fillet Whole Wheat Penne with Spinach (page 195)
WEDNESDAY LUNCH	Dillicious Spinach Frittata (page 128) Mixed fruit salad of cantaloupe, berries and mango
THURSDAY DINNER	Beef and Broccoli with Barley (page 219) Green tea
FRIDAY LUNCH	Tuna salad (using light canned tuna) with green onion served in an orange bell pepper half Low-fat yogurt topped with diced kiwifruit Sparkling water with lemon and lime

Shopping List for Two

This list includes all of the food necessary to prepare the recipes in the meal plan above. You will have extra produce and a stocked pantry (see page 124) to use in the rest of your daily meals.

Produce

- 1 package frozen spinach
- 4 orange bell peppers
- 1 head broccoli
- 1 bunch green onions
- 1 head garlic
- 1 gingerroot
- 1 head romaine lettuce
- 1 bunch fresh cilantro
- 1 bunch fresh dill
- 1 lemon
- 2 limes
- 4 oranges
- 1 container berries of your choice
- ½ cantaloupe
- 2 kiwifruit
- 1 mango

Meat, Fish and Dairy

- 8 oz (250 g) lean beef (such as tenderloin or sirloin)
- 7 oz (200 g) grilled turkey breast slices (or you can buy raw and grill it yourself)
- 2 salmon fillets (each about 5 oz/150 g)
- 1 can light tuna
- 6 large omega-3 eggs
- 1 quart (1 L) milk
- 1 container low-fat plain yogurt
- 4 slices Swiss cheese

Grocery

- 1 loaf whole-grain bread
- Whole wheat penne or other whole-grain or bean pasta
- Barley
- 1 can chickpeas (any size)
- Grated Parmesan cheese
- 1 jar sun-dried tomatoes
- Olive oil
- Extra virgin olive oil
- Mustard
- Soy sauce
- Chili powder
- Wasabi paste
- Ready-to-use reduced-sodium beef broth
- Green tea
- Sparkling water

Week 2	
MONDAY LUNCH	Chicken and Almond Lettuce Wraps (page 209) Raw broccoli with White Bean Dip (page 227) Green tea
TUESDAY DINNER	Rainbow Trout Packets (page 203) Carrot Fries (page 185)
WEDNESDAY LUNCH	Leftover rainbow trout from Tuesday night's dinner (enjoy it cold) Mango Spinach Salad (page 158)
THURSDAY DINNER	Turkey Fajitas (page 212) Sparkling water with lemon and lime
FRIDAY LUNCH	Crustless Quiche (page 199) Salad of baby spinach topped with berries and drizzled with a dressing of olive oil, lemon juice, salt and pepper

Shopping List for Two

This list includes all of the food necessary to prepare the recipes in the meal plan above, aside from some staples you should still have on hand from last week. You will have extra produce and a stocked pantry (see page 124) to use in the rest of your daily meals.

Produce

- 1 bag frozen green peas
- 1 bag frozen corn kernels
- 2 orange bell peppers
- 2 red bell peppers
- 1 or 2 jalapeño peppers
- 1 head broccoli
- 4 carrots
- 1 head garlic
- 1 Spanish or Vidalia onion
- 1 yellow onion
- 8 green onions
- 8 oz (250 g) kale
- 1 head romaine lettuce
- 6 oz (175 g) baby spinach
- 1 bunch cilantro
- 1 bunch parsley
- 1 bunch tarragon
- 3 lemons
- 4 limes
- 1 large and 2 small oranges
- 1 container berries of your choice
- 1 mango

Meat, Fish and Dairy

- ○ 20 oz (600 g) boneless skinless chicken breasts
- ○ 1½ lbs (750 g) boneless skinless turkey breasts (or chicken breasts)
- ○ 20 oz (600 g) rainbow trout fillets
- ○ 6 large omega-3 eggs
- ○ 1 quart (1 L) milk
- ○ 1 container sour cream
- ○ 1 package shredded Cheddar cheese (or 1 brick, to shred your own)

Miscellaneous

- ○ Eight 12-inch (30 cm) whole-grain flour or corn tortillas
- ○ One 19-oz (540 mL) can or two 14- or 15-oz (398 or 425 mL) cans cannellini (white kidney) beans
- ○ 1 can black beans (any size)
- ○ Sliced almonds
- ○ Natural almond or peanut butter
- ○ Green pumpkin seeds (pepitas)
- ○ 1 jar sun-dried tomatoes
- ○ Paprika (if using on the Carrot Fries)
- ○ Ground cumin
- ○ Hot pepper sauce
- ○ Liquid honey
- ○ Unseasoned rice vinegar
- ○ Apple cider vinegar
- ○ Ready-to-use chicken broth
- ○ Salsa
- ○ Sparkling water

Pantry and Freezer Lists

Shopping for and preparing foods ahead of time can make it easier to follow the Eyefoods Plan. Stock your pantry and freezer with these ingredients to make prepping eye-healthy meals quick and simple.

Pantry List

- ○ Almonds
- ○ Cashews
- ○ Walnuts
- ○ Natural almond or peanut butter
- ○ Flax seeds
- ○ Green pumpkin seeds (pepitas)
- ○ Sunflower seeds
- ○ Dried apricots
- ○ Dried goji berries
- ○ Sugar-free steel-cut oats
- ○ Black beans
- ○ Cannellini (white kidney) beans
- ○ Chickpeas
- ○ Romano beans
- ○ Pumpkin purée (not pie filling)
- ○ Olive oil
- ○ Extra-virgin olive oil
- ○ Apple cider vinegar
- ○ Balsamic vinegar
- ○ Unseasoned rice vinegar
- ○ Wine vinegar
- ○ Liquid honey
- ○ Pure maple syrup
- ○ Green tea

Freezer List

- ○ Green beans
- ○ Green peas
- ○ Spinach
- ○ Berries
- ○ Sliced mango
- ○ Lean cuts of beef
- ○ Chicken breast
- ○ Turkey breast
- ○ Rainbow trout fillets
- ○ Salmon fillets

Pro Tip

Prepare eyefoods staples — slice orange bell peppers, chop broccoli, chop kale and spinach, hard-cook eggs, slice kiwifruit — and keep them in airtight containers in the fridge, making them easy to grab and go or prep meals with.

PART 3

Recipes for Healthy Eyes

Breakfasts

Breakfast is the most important meal of the day, and what better way to start your day than with an eye-healthy meal? The recipes in this section are filled with eye-friendly nutrients, including beta-carotene, lutein, zeaxanthin, vitamin C, vitamin E and zinc. Many eyefoods, including eggs, spinach, nuts, berries and citrus fruits, are great additions to breakfast recipes.

Orange Pepper, Spinach and Sun-Dried Tomato Frittata...............127

Dillicious Spinach Frittata......................................128

Perfect Poached Eggs...129

Eggs Benny with Roasted Pepper Coulis 129

Kale and Sweet Potato Hash 130

Pumpkin Savory Loaf 131

Green Smoothie Bowl..132

Chocolate Smoothie Bowl 133

Eyefoods Fruit Salad 134

Kiwi, Mango and Blackberry Fruit Bowl..........................134

Orange Pepper, Spinach and Sun-Dried Tomato Frittata

EYE NUTRIENTS: Lutein, zeaxanthin, vitamin C, vitamin E, zinc, omega-3s (ALA and DHA)

MAKES 2 SERVINGS

A frittata is an Italian egg dish that can be enjoyed for breakfast, lunch or dinner. A quick meal, it can be served hot or prepared ahead of time and served cold.

TIPS: If you have an ovenproof skillet, you can also cook the frittata under the broiler. Preheat the broiler, then, after pouring in the egg mixture in step 3, broil for 3 minutes or until the top of the frittata is set.

Here are some fun ways to serve a frittata:

- **Breakfast:** Make a breakfast sandwich with whole-grain toast, ½ frittata, ½ avocado, sliced or mashed, and a slice of tomato.

- **Lunch:** Cut the frittata into quarters and, serving 2 quarters per person, create asparagus frittata towers by alternating layers of frittata and steamed asparagus.

- **Dinner:** Serve the frittata with a side of kale chips (see recipes, pages 223–225).

3	large omega-3 eggs	3
1 tbsp	chopped fresh parsley	15 mL
Pinch	salt	Pinch
Pinch	freshly ground black pepper	Pinch
1 tbsp	milk	15 mL
1 tbsp	olive oil	15 mL
½ cup	finely chopped orange bell pepper	125 mL
¼ cup	chopped drained oil-packed sun-dried tomatoes	60 mL
¼ cup	frozen chopped spinach	60 mL

1. In a bowl, whisk together eggs, parsley, salt, pepper and milk; set aside.

2. In a small nonstick skillet, heat oil over medium-high heat. Add orange pepper and sun-dried tomatoes; cook, stirring, for 1 minute. Add spinach and cook, stirring, until thawed.

3. Reduce heat to low and pour in egg mixture, ensuring that vegetables and eggs are evenly distributed in the pan. Cook, without stirring, for about 5 minutes or until top of frittata begins to set (ensure that the bottom does not burn; if it looks like it is starting to, flip it earlier). Invert a plate over top of pan, flip pan and frittata over onto plate, then slide frittata back into pan. Cook for 1 to 2 minutes or until bottom is set.

Eyefood Focus

The Eyefoods Plan recommends eating 4 eggs, with yolks, per week. The yolk is full of important eye nutrients, including vitamin E, lutein, zinc and the omega-3 fatty acid DHA. Studies show that consuming 1 egg per day raises the lutein level in your body without increasing your serum cholesterol.

Dillicious Spinach Frittata

EYE NUTRIENTS: Lutein, zeaxanthin, vitamin C, vitamin E, zinc, omega-3s (ALA and DHA)

This egg dish is one of the first eyefoods recipes I created. It quickly became a staple in my home, and I have introduced it to many friends and family throughout the years. Eggs, orange peppers, green onions and spinach make this versatile dish a lutein and zeaxanthin powerhouse.

TIPS: If you have an ovenproof skillet, you can also cook the frittata under the broiler. Preheat the broiler, then, after pouring in the egg mixture in step 3, broil for 3 minutes or until the top of the frittata is set.

The frittata can also be enjoyed at room temperature or even cold the next day.

When serving omelets and frittatas to kids, make them fun by creating faces using healthy vegetables such as tomatoes, asparagus and peas. Use spinach or lettuce for hair.

Eyefood Focus

Cooking spinach and orange peppers helps break down their cell walls and improves your body's uptake of lutein and zeaxanthin.

3	large omega-3 eggs	3
1 tbsp	chopped fresh dill	15 mL
Pinch	salt	Pinch
Pinch	freshly ground black pepper	Pinch
1 tbsp	milk	15 mL
1 tbsp	olive oil	15 mL
1	green onion, chopped	1
½ cup	finely chopped orange bell pepper	125 mL
¼ cup	frozen chopped spinach	60 mL

1. In a bowl, whisk together eggs, dill, salt, pepper and milk; set aside.

2. In a small nonstick skillet, heat oil over medium-high heat. Add green onion and orange pepper; cook, stirring, for 1 minute. Add spinach and cook, stirring, until thawed.

3. Reduce heat to low and pour in egg mixture, ensuring that vegetables and eggs are evenly distributed in the pan. Cook, without stirring, for about 5 minutes or until top of frittata begins to set (ensure that the bottom does not burn; if it looks like it is starting to, flip it earlier). Invert a plate over top of pan, flip pan and frittata over onto plate, then slide frittata back into pan. Cook for 1 to 2 minutes or until bottom is set.

Perfect Poached Eggs

EYE NUTRIENTS: Lutein, vitamin E, zinc, omega-3s (ALA and DHA)

Poaching is one of the most nutritious ways to prepare eggs. Poached eggs are great served atop a piece of whole-grain toast or, even better, a bed of spinach. Here is a tried-and-true method for perfect poached eggs.

Eyefood Focus

There is less lutein in eggs than in leafy green vegetables, such as spinach and kale, but the lutein in eggs is highly bioavailable and is absorbed well by our bodies.

	Large omega-3 eggs	
1 tbsp	white vinegar	15 mL

1. Fill a large saucepan three-quarters full with water. Add vinegar and bring to a simmer over high heat.

2. Meanwhile, crack each egg into its own ramekin or small bowl.

3. When water comes to a simmer, reduce heat to maintain a gentle simmer. Using a slotted spoon, stir water clockwise, creating a swirl. While the water is swirling, slowly pour each egg into the center of the pan. Cook for $3\frac{1}{2}$ minutes for a soft, runny yolk or 5 minutes for a hard yolk. If the water starts to boil too hard, reduce the heat.

4. Using a slotted spoon, remove each egg from the water and gently place them on a plate lined with a paper towel to absorb the excess water. Serve hot.

Eggs Benny with Roasted Pepper Coulis

EYE NUTRIENTS: Lutein, zeaxanthin, vitamin C, vitamin E, zinc, omega-3s (ALA and DHA)

MAKES 2 SERVINGS

Eggs Benedict is a brunch staple, and this eye-healthy recipe is perfect for vegetarians or anyone watching their meat intake. Impress your family and friends with this nutritious take on a classic dish.

4	large omega-3 eggs	4
2	whole-grain English muffins, split	2
1 cup	packed baby spinach or pea shoots	250 mL
1	avocado, sliced	1
4 tbsp	Roasted Pepper Coulis (page 187)	60 mL

1. Poach eggs, following the instructions in the recipe above.

2. Meanwhile, toast English muffins.

3. Place one-quarter of the spinach on each English muffin half. Add one-quarter of the avocado slices. Top each with a poached egg and drizzle with 1 tbsp (15 mL) coulis.

Kale and Sweet Potato Hash

EYE NUTRIENTS: Beta-carotene, lutein, zeaxanthin, vitamin C, vitamin E, zinc, omega-3s (ALA and DHA)

MAKES 1 SERVING

If you roast your sweet potatoes ahead of time and keep chopped prewashed kale in the fridge, you can prepare this one-dish breakfast very quickly.

TIP: Buy a large bunch of kale at the beginning of the week. Wash it thoroughly and dry it in a salad spinner. Wrap kale in a tea towel or paper towel, place it in a plastic bag, and store it in the fridge, ready to use during the week.

Eyefood Focus

Eggs are considered a complete protein, containing all nine essential amino acids, the building blocks of protein.

1 tbsp	olive oil	15 mL
1 cup	chopped trimmed kale	250 mL
1 cup	chopped tomatoes	250 mL
½ cup	roasted cubed sweet potatoes (see tip, page 133)	125 mL
1	large omega-3 egg	1
	Salt and freshly ground black pepper	

1. In a skillet, heat oil over medium heat. Add kale and tomatoes; cook, stirring, for 3 to 4 minutes or until kale is wilted but still vibrant in color. Add sweet potatoes and cook, stirring, for 1 to 2 minutes or until warmed through.

2. Spread vegetables to cover bottom of skillet evenly. Crack egg onto the mixture. Cook, without stirring, for about 3 minutes for a softly set egg, or to desired doneness. (If you like the top of your egg to cook more, you may need to cover with a lid for the last 30 seconds of cooking.)

Pumpkin Savory Loaf

EYE NUTRIENTS: Beta-carotene, fiber, omega-3s (ALA and DHA)

MAKES 8 SERVINGS

Enjoy a slice of this nutritious loaf in place of toast alongside any egg dish. The pumpkin makes it a great source of beta-carotene, and the oats and whole wheat flour add to the fiber content.

TIP: Store the cooled loaf in an airtight container at room temperature for up to 5 days.

Eyefood Focus

Omega-3 eggs come from hens that are fed a diet high in flax seeds, which contain the plant-based omega-3 fatty acid ALA (alpha-linolenic acid). The hen converts some of the ALA into DHA (docosahexaenoic acid), which is normally found in fish, and both ALA and DHA are transferred into the egg yolk. DHA is abundant in the cells of our retina.

- Preheat oven to 350°F (180°C)
- Blender or immersion blender
- Electric mixer
- 9- by 5-inch (23 by 12.5 cm) loaf pan, greased with olive oil

1 tbsp	olive oil	15 mL
1 cup	chopped onion	250 mL
1½ cups	whole wheat flour	375 mL
½ cup	large-flake (old-fashioned) rolled oats	125 mL
½ cup	natural wheat bran	125 mL
2 tbsp	chopped fresh sage	30 mL
2 tsp	baking powder	10 mL
½ tsp	baking soda	2 mL
Pinch	salt	Pinch
2	large omega-3 eggs	2
1 cup	pumpkin purée (not pie filling)	250 mL
½ cup	milk	125 mL
¼ cup	olive oil	60 mL
¼ cup	packed brown sugar	60 mL

1. In a medium skillet, heat 1 tbsp (15 mL) oil over medium-high heat. Add onion and cook, stirring, for 5 to 7 minutes or until tender. Remove from heat and let cool for 10 minutes.

2. Transfer cooled onion to blender (or transfer to a small bowl and use an immersion blender) and purée until smooth. Set aside.

3. In a medium bowl, whisk together flour, oats, bran, sage, baking powder, baking soda and salt.

4. In a large bowl, using an electric mixer, beat eggs, pumpkin, onion purée, milk and ¼ cup (60 mL) oil. Add brown sugar and mix well. Add dry ingredients and, using a wooden spoon, stir gently just until moistened.

5. Pour batter into prepared pan and smooth top.

6. Bake in preheated oven for about 1 hour or until a toothpick inserted in the center comes out clean. Let cool in pan on a wire rack for 20 minutes. Remove from pan and let cool completely.

Green Smoothie Bowl

EYE NUTRIENTS: Lutein, zeaxanthin, vitamin C, omega-3s (ALA)

MAKES 1 SERVING

A smoothie bowl is a twist on a traditional smoothie. It is thicker, and you eat it with a spoon instead of drinking it with a straw. Think of the smoothie as the milk and the toppings as the cereal. It is a nutrient power punch that is great for breakfast or after a workout.

VARIATION: Other great toppings include rolled oats, slivered almonds, chopped walnuts or dried apricots.

Eyefood Focus

Goji berries are native to parts of Asia and are one of the few food sources of zeaxanthin. They are typically found dried, in packages or in the bulk food section of your supermarket.

• **Blender**

¼ to ½ cup	coconut water	60 to 125 mL
½	banana, sliced	½
¼	avocado	¼
1 cup	packed chopped trimmed spinach	250 mL
½ cup	frozen pineapple chunks	125 mL
1 tsp	matcha powder	5 mL

Toppings

1 tbsp	dried goji berries	15 mL
1 tbsp	chia seeds	15 mL
1 tbsp	hemp seeds	15 mL
	Sliced starfruit, kiwifruit or berries	
	Shredded coconut	

1. In blender, combine ¼ cup (60 mL) coconut water, banana, avocado, spinach, pineapple and matcha; purée until smooth, adding more coconut water as needed for the desired consistency.

2. Spoon smoothie into your favorite dessert or cereal bowl. Add toppings decoratively, with seeds on one side and fruit on the other. Serve immediately.

Chocolate Smoothie Bowl

EYE NUTRIENTS: Beta-carotene, lutein, zeaxanthin, vitamin C, vitamin E, omega-3s (ALA)

MAKES 1 SERVING

Don't let the kale and sweet potatoes fool you — all you can taste in this delicious and nutritious smoothie bowl is chocolate. You won't believe it's a healthy choice.

TIP: Roast a pan of sweet potatoes at the beginning of the week. Peel and cut sweet potatoes into ½-inch (1 cm) cubes and place on a rimmed baking sheet. Drizzle with olive oil, season with salt and toss to coat, then spread out into a single layer. Roast in a 400°F (200°C) oven for about 25 minutes or until tender. Let cool. Store in an airtight container in the refrigerator for up to 1 week.

Eyefood Focus

Eat three servings of fruit per day. The best choices include kiwifruit, berries and citrus fruit.

- **Blender**

¼ to ½ cup	unsweetened almond milk or water	60 to 125 mL
½	frozen banana	½
1 cup	packed chopped trimmed kale	250 mL
¼ cup	roasted cubed sweet potato (see tip)	60 mL
¼ cup	frozen blueberries	60 mL
1 tbsp	unsweetened cocoa powder	15 mL

Toppings

1 tbsp	chopped walnuts	15 mL
1 tbsp	hemp seeds	15 mL
	Sliced strawberries	

1. In blender, combine ¼ cup (60 mL) almond milk, banana, kale, sweet potatoes, blueberries and cocoa; purée until smooth, adding more milk as needed for the desired consistency.

2. Spoon smoothie into your favorite dessert or cereal bowl. Add toppings decoratively, with nuts and seeds on one side and strawberries on the other. Serve immediately.

Eyefoods Fruit Salad

EYE NUTRIENTS: Beta-carotene, zeaxanthin, vitamin C, fiber

Kiwifruit is the vitamin C powerhouse of this visually appealing fruit salad, while cantaloupe adds a dash of beta-carotene. The goji berries contribute both zeaxanthin and a pleasant texture.

TIP: A fruit salad makes a great breakfast, snack or even dessert. Make a big bowl and store it, covered, in your fridge for up to 3 days.

½	cantaloupe	½
2	kiwifruit, peeled	2
	Juice of 1 lime	
1 tbsp	pure maple syrup	15 mL
1 cup	seedless red grapes	250 mL
¼ cup	dried goji berries	60 mL

1. Use a melon baller to make cantaloupe balls, reserving trimmings for another use.

2. Cut kiwis lengthwise into quarters, then cut each quarter crosswise into 4 pieces.

3. In a small bowl, combine lime juice and maple syrup.

4. In serving bowl, combine melon balls, kiwis and grapes. Pour juice mixture over fruit and stir gently to coat. Serve garnished with goji berries.

Kiwi, Mango and Blackberry Fruit Bowl

EYE NUTRIENTS: Vitamin C, vitamin E, fiber

This is one of my all-time favorite fruit combinations. I love the zestiness of the blackberries and kiwi, combined with the sweetness of the mango. So vibrant in color, it looks great in a bowl.

6	kiwifruit, peeled and sliced	6
1	mango, chopped	1
1 cup	blackberries	250 mL
1 tbsp	pure maple syrup or liquid honey (optional)	15 mL
1 tbsp	freshly squeezed lemon juice	15 mL

1. In a bowl, combine kiwis, mango and blackberries. Add maple syrup, if desired, and lemon juice; stir gently to coat.

> **Eyefood Focus**
>
> Mangos are a source of vitamin E, which is more typically found in oils and other fats. Eating mangos is a great low-fat way to increase your vitamin E intake.

Smoothies and Juices

Smoothies and juices are an excellent way to get the most important nutrients for eye health in a deliciously drinkable form. If you drink one of these beverages every day, you will consistently consume high amounts of lutein, zeaxanthin and vitamin C. And what better way to brighten your day? Delicious and packed with nutrients, these drinks are beloved by both kids and adults alike. So pull that blender or juicer out of your cupboard and keep it on your countertop!

What's the Difference Between Smoothies and Juices?. 136
Eyefoods-Infused Water 137

Green Smoothies

Not-So-Green Smoothie
  for Beginners. 138
Dr. Barb's Green Smoothie. 139
Berry Banana Green Smoothie 140
Peach Grape Green Smoothie. 140
Vanilla Pear Green Smoothie. 141
Melon Mint Green Smoothie 141
Mango, Mint and Lime
  Green Smoothie 142
Kiwi Mango Green Smoothie. 142
Orange Kiwi Green Smoothie 143
Tropical Eye Power Green Smoothie. . .143
Banana Matcha Green Smoothie. 144

Chocolate Goji Berry
  Green Smoothie 144
Melon Matcha Green Smoothie. 145

Fruit and Veggie Smoothies

Strawberry, Watermelon and Mint
  Smoothie 146
Coconut Berry Smoothie 146
Goji Berry Smoothie 147
Peach, Pineapple and Pepper
  Smoothie 147
Carrot Mango Smoothie 148
Pumpkin Pie Smoothie 148
Cantaloupe Drinkable Yogurt 149

Juices

Beta-Carotene Blast 149
Citrus Zinger. 150
Pear, Ginger and Mint Juice. 150

What's the Difference Between Smoothies and Juices?

Smoothies

Smoothies are prepared in a blender. To make a smoothie, fruits and/or vegetables are blended with water or another liquid until the mixture is smooth and drinkable. Because they use the whole fruit or vegetable, smoothies contain fiber, which is a necessary part of an eye-healthy diet. Fiber also helps maintain a healthy digestive system and will make you feel full sooner and stay full longer.

One great thing about making your own smoothies is that you control the amount of liquid you put in, and thus the consistency of your creation. If you prefer to eat your food with a spoon rather than drink it, a smoothie bowl may be for you. Any smoothie recipe in this chapter can be transformed into a smoothie bowl — simply reduce the amount of liquid in the recipe. You'll also find a couple of smoothie bowl recipes in the previous chapter.

This chapter includes a good selection of tasty green smoothies, as well as recipes featuring other eye-healthy vegetables and fruits. The Eyefoods Plan recommends eating 1 cup (250 mL) or one handful of raw leafy green vegetables per day and three $\frac{1}{2}$-cup (125 mL) servings of fruit per day. Enjoying a green smoothie every day will ensure that you meet these recommendations and nourish your eyes with high amounts of lutein and other eye nutrients.

Smoothies have the highest nutritional content if consumed immediately after they are prepared. However, you can store them in an airtight jar, filled to the top, in the refrigerator for up to 2 days. Adding lemon or lime juice and filling the jar to the top will help prevent oxidation and keep the nutrient level high. Before drinking leftovers, shake well.

Juices

Juices are prepared with a juicer, which extracts the liquid from fruits and vegetables. This liquid contains all of the nutrients that were present in the whole produce, but does not contain any fiber. If you are already consuming a lot of fiber, including juices in your diet may be a good option for you, as the body absorbs nutrients from juice faster than from smoothies, helping you feel energized. Because the solid part of the produce is discarded, a large quantity of fruits and vegetables are needed to make each serving of juice, meaning you reap the benefits of a higher concentration of nutrients than you can get in a smoothie or from eating whole fruits and vegetables.

Juice is most nutritious if enjoyed immediately, but it can be refrigerated in a glass jar, filled to the top and covered, for up to 1 day.

Eyefoods-Infused Water

Stay hydrated with eyefoods-infused water! Follow these simple steps to create refreshing drinks for the whole family.

1. Choose a glass pitcher and add a handful of chopped herbs or spices from the list below.

2. Choose one or two fruits and/or veggies from the list below. Slice and add to the pitcher.

3. Fill the pitcher with water and chill in the fridge for at least 2 hours to allow the flavors to infuse into the water.

Herbs and Spices	Fruits	Vegetables
Basil	Blueberries	Cucumber
Ginger	Kiwifruit	Fennel
Mint	Lemon	
Rosemary	Lime	
	Mango	
	Orange	
	Peach	
	Raspberries	
	Strawberries	
	Watermelon	

Infused water will last up to 3 days, but the fruit and veggies may get waterlogged within a day. If you haven't finished it all in 24 hours, strain out the produce and return the water to the fridge.

Not-So-Green Smoothie for Beginners

EYE NUTRIENTS: Lutein, zeaxanthin, vitamin C

MAKES 2 SERVINGS

Sweetened with orange juice and maple syrup, this smoothie appeals to most palates — and you can't taste the spinach one bit! It's a good choice if you have a sweet tooth.

TIP: In place of frozen, use fresh peaches when they are in season. If using fresh peaches, you will need to reduce the amount of orange juice to keep your smoothie thick.

Eyefood Focus

Maple syrup is a source of vitamin E. Use maple syrup in place of sugar to sweeten recipes, but remember that it is still a sugar and high in calories, and use it in small amounts.

• Blender

1 cup	orange juice (approx.)	250 mL
1 tbsp	pure maple syrup	15 mL
2 cups	frozen sliced peaches	500 mL
1 cup	packed baby spinach	250 mL

1. In blender, combine orange juice, maple syrup, peaches and spinach; blend until smooth. If a thinner consistency is desired, blend in orange juice as needed.

Dr. Barb's Green Smoothie

EYE NUTRIENTS: Lutein, zeaxanthin, vitamin C

This tried-and-true recipe was the first smoothie the eyefoods team created. It became a quick hit, and we served it at many eye health events and conferences. Make it a staple in your eye-healthy diet.

TIPS: The flavor of this smoothie will vary depending on how sweet the grapes and kiwis are. If they are quite sweet, add the lime juice. If they are tart, omit it.

If your kiwis are quite sweet, increase the amount of kiwi in the smoothie and decrease the amount of grapes (or banana) accordingly, for more eye nutrients.

VARIATION: Replace the grapes with 1 banana, broken into chunks. Include the optional lime juice to reduce oxidation (browning) of the banana if you don't plan on drinking all of the smoothie right away.

• **Blender**

1 cup	water (approx.)	250 mL
2	kiwifruit, peeled and quartered	2
2 cups	packed chopped trimmed kale	500 mL
1 cup	seedless green grapes	250 mL
	Juice of 1 lime (optional)	

1. In blender, combine water, kiwis, kale and grapes; blend until smooth. Taste and add lime juice, if desired (see tip). If a thinner consistency is desired, blend in more water as needed.

Berry Banana Green Smoothie

EYE NUTRIENTS: Lutein, zeaxanthin, vitamin C, fiber

MAKES 1 TO
2 SERVINGS

Berries and bananas are a classic smoothie combination, and the addition of kale makes it even more eye-healthy. Thanks to the vanilla and coconut or almond milk, you'll think you're drinking a milkshake!

Eyefood Focus

A great source of antioxidants, berries are also low in calories and high in fiber, making them an important part of the Eyefoods Plan. Enjoy them year-round, either fresh or frozen.

- **Blender**

¾ cup	unsweetened coconut milk beverage or plain almond milk (approx.)	175 mL
1 tsp	vanilla extract	5 mL
1	small banana, broken into chunks	1
1 cup	packed baby kale	250 mL
¾ cup	frozen raspberries	175 mL

Optional Add-Ins

1	scoop protein powder	1
1 tbsp	hemp seeds	15 mL

1. In blender, combine coconut milk, vanilla, banana, kale, raspberries and any desired add-ins; blend until smooth. If a thinner consistency is desired, blend in more coconut milk as needed.

Peach Grape Green Smoothie

EYE NUTRIENTS: Lutein, zeaxanthin, vitamin C

MAKES 1 TO
2 SERVINGS

Enjoy a taste of summer year-round with this delicious creation that uses frozen peaches.

- **Blender**

½ cup	water (approx.)	125 mL
1 cup	packed chopped trimmed kale or spinach	250 mL
¾ cup	sliced frozen peaches	175 mL
½ cup	seedless green grapes	125 mL

1. In blender, combine water, kale, peaches and grapes; blend until smooth. If a thinner consistency is desired, blend in more water as needed.

Vanilla Pear Green Smoothie

EYE NUTRIENTS: Lutein, zeaxanthin, vitamin C, fiber

MAKES 1 TO 2 SERVINGS

This sweet, nutritious smoothie is a real treat — you'll find it hard to believe you're not drinking a milkshake.

TIP: If you have a high-speed blender, there's no need to trim and chop the kale before making your smoothie. Use 1 average-size leaf with the stem (about 0.9 oz/25 g) and simply add it to the blender whole.

• **Blender**

1 cup	water (approx.)	250 mL
½ cup	unsweetened plain almond milk	125 mL
1 tsp	vanilla extract	5 mL
1	Bosc pear, cut into chunks	1
1	banana, broken into chunks	1
1 cup	packed chopped trimmed kale	250 mL
⅛ tsp	ground cinnamon	0.5 mL

1. In blender, combine water, almond milk, vanilla, pear, banana, kale and cinnamon; blend until smooth. If a thinner consistency is desired, blend in more water as needed.

Melon Mint Green Smoothie

EYE NUTRIENTS: Lutein, zeaxanthin, vitamin C

MAKES 1 TO 2 SERVINGS

At an optometry conference in Ottawa, Canada, Dr. Barb and I held a smoothie challenge between this recipe and Dr. Barb's Green Smoothie (page 139). It was a close competition, but this smoothie was the favorite of the day.

TIP: If you are not consuming the smoothie immediately, lime juice is essential to reduce browning of the banana.

• **Blender**

1 cup	water (approx.)	250 mL
	Juice of ½ lime (optional)	
15	fresh mint leaves	15
1	banana, broken into chunks	1
1½ cups	packed chopped trimmed kale	375 mL
1 cup	chopped honeydew melon	250 mL

1. In blender, combine water, lime juice (if using), mint, banana, kale and melon; blend until smooth. If a thinner consistency is desired, blend in more water as needed.

Mango, Mint and Lime Green Smoothie

EYE NUTRIENTS: Lutein, zeaxanthin, vitamin C, vitamin E

MAKES 1 TO 2 SERVINGS

Mango is one of my favorite fruits, and it pairs wonderfully with mint in this creamy treat.

- **Blender**

1 cup	unsweetened coconut milk beverage (approx.)	250 mL
	Juice of ½ lime	
5	fresh mint leaves	5
1 cup	packed chopped trimmed kale or spinach	250 mL
1 cup	frozen mango chunks	250 mL

1. In blender, combine coconut milk, lime juice, mint, kale and mango; blend until smooth. If a thinner consistency is desired, blend in more coconut milk as needed.

Kiwi Mango Green Smoothie

EYE NUTRIENTS: Lutein, zeaxanthin, vitamin C, vitamin E, fiber

MAKES 3 TO 4 SERVINGS

A kiwifruit provides more vitamin C than any other fruit — more than twice as much as an orange — and this smoothie ups the ante with kale, another great source of this vital antioxidant.

TIP: If you have a high-speed blender, there's no need to trim and chop the kale before making your smoothie. For each cup (250 mL) of kale called for, use 1 average-size leaf with the stem (about 0.9 oz/25 g) and simply add it to the blender whole.

- **Blender**

1½ cups	water (approx.)	375 mL
4	yellow kiwifruit, peeled and quartered	4
2	green kiwifruit, peeled and quartered	2
3 cups	packed chopped trimmed kale	750 mL
1 cup	frozen mango chunks	250 mL

1. In blender, combine water, yellow kiwis, green kiwis, kale and mango; blend until smooth. If a thinner consistency is desired, blend in more water as needed.

Orange Kiwi Green Smoothie

EYE NUTRIENTS: Lutein, zeaxanthin, vitamin C, fiber

MAKES 1 TO 2 SERVINGS

With kale, kiwis and oranges, this smoothie is a vitamin C powerhouse.

TIP: Use ripe kiwis for a sweeter flavor.

- Blender
- Fine rasp grater (such as a Microplane)

1 cup	water (approx.)	250 mL
2 cups	packed chopped trimmed kale	500 mL
2	kiwifruit, peeled and quartered	2
2	oranges	2

1. In blender, combine water, kale and kiwis.

2. Using the fine grater, grate orange zest from both oranges into blender. Using a sharp knife, cut off orange peel and pith (white part) of both oranges and discard; add orange flesh to blender.

3. Blend until smooth. If a thinner consistency is desired, blend in more water as needed.

Tropical Eye Power Green Smoothie

EYE NUTRIENTS: Lutein, zeaxanthin, vitamin C, vitamin E, omega-3s (ALA)

MAKES 1 SERVING

In addition to nourishing your eyes, the coconut water in this refreshing treat will replenish much-needed electrolytes after a run or workout.

Eyefood Focus

In addition to being a great source of healthy fats, including plant-based omega-3 fatty acids, avocado contains a small amount of lutein.

- Blender

¾ cup	coconut water (approx.)	175 mL
1 cup	packed chopped trimmed spinach or kale	250 mL
¾ cup	frozen mango chunks	175 mL
¼ cup	chopped pineapple	60 mL

Optional Add-Ins

¼	avocado, sliced	¼
1 tbsp	plain Greek yogurt	15 mL
1 tbsp	coconut oil	15 mL

1. In blender, combine coconut water, spinach, mango, pineapple and any desired add-ins; blend until smooth. If a thinner consistency is desired, blend in more coconut water as needed.

Banana Matcha Green Smoothie

EYE NUTRIENTS: Lutein, vitamin C

The green tea in this smoothie provides an antioxidant boost, and it tastes so good, you won't believe how good it is for you. It is best enjoyed immediately, to reap the benefits of the antioxidants.

TIP: Matcha green tea powder can be found at most health food stores and specialty tea shops. If you don't have matcha, you can replace it with regular green tea. Use ¾ cup (175 mL) brewed green tea in place of the matcha powder, hot water and cold water.

- **Blender**

1 tsp	matcha powder	5 mL
2 tbsp	hot water (not boiling)	30 mL
¾ cup	cold water (approx.)	175 mL
	Juice of 1 lime	
2	large ripe bananas, broken into chunks	2
3 cups	packed baby spinach	750 mL

1. In a small bowl, whisk matcha with hot water until dissolved. Pour into blender.

2. Add cold water, lime juice, bananas and spinach to blender and blend until smooth. If a thinner consistency is desired, blend in more cold water as needed.

Chocolate Goji Berry Green Smoothie

EYE NUTRIENTS: Lutein, zeaxanthin, vitamin C

Goji berry powder provides loads of zeaxanthin in this delicious chocolate smoothie.

TIPS: For the greens, try kale, spinach or dandelion greens.

Goji berry powder can be found at health food stores.

- **Blender**

¾ cup	unsweetened coconut milk beverage or plain almond milk (approx.)	175 mL
1	frozen banana, broken into chunks	1
1 cup	packed chopped trimmed leafy greens	250 mL
1 tbsp	goji berry powder	15 mL
1 tbsp	unsweetened cocoa powder	15 mL
½ cup	ice cubes	125 mL

1. In blender, combine coconut milk, banana, greens, goji berry powder, cocoa and ice; blend until smooth. If a thinner consistency is desired, blend in more coconut milk as needed.

Melon Matcha Green Smoothie

EYE NUTRIENTS: Lutein, zeaxanthin, vitamin C

MAKES 2 SERVINGS

Matcha contains even more antioxidants than regular green tea, but you'll want to enjoy this smoothie immediately for the most benefits.

TIPS: Matcha green tea powder can be found at most health food stores and specialty tea shops. If you don't have matcha, you can replace it with regular green tea. Use 1 cup (250 mL) brewed green tea in place of the matcha powder and hot water.

If you have a high-speed blender, there's no need to trim and chop the kale before making your smoothie. For each cup (250 mL) of kale called for, use 1 average-size leaf with the stem (about 0.9 oz/25 g) and simply add it to the blender whole.

- **Blender**

1 tsp	matcha powder	5 mL
1 cup	hot water (not boiling)	250 mL
3 cups	packed chopped trimmed kale	750 mL
1½ cups	chopped honeydew melon	375 mL
½ cup	ice cubes	125 mL
	Cold water (optional)	

1. In a small bowl, whisk matcha with hot water until dissolved. Pour into blender.

2. Add kale, melon and ice to blender and blend until smooth. If a thinner consistency is desired, blend in cold water as needed.

> **Eyefood Focus**
> Green tea has been shown to help decrease the symptoms of dry eye syndrome.

Strawberry, Watermelon and Mint Smoothie

EYE NUTRIENTS: Vitamin C

> ### MAKES 1 TO 2 SERVINGS

This tasty red smoothie is refreshing on a hot summer day.

TIP: For a more liquid consistency, you can use more watermelon.

- **Blender**

½ cup	coconut water (approx.)	125 mL
	Juice of ½ lime	
10	fresh mint leaves	10
1 cup	frozen strawberries	250 mL
1 cup	diced watermelon	250 mL
¼ cup	sliced peeled cucumber	60 mL

1. In blender, combine coconut water, lime juice, mint, strawberries, watermelon and cucumber; blend until smooth. If a thinner consistency is desired, blend in more coconut water as needed.

Coconut Berry Smoothie

EYE NUTRIENTS: Vitamin C, omega-3s (ALA), fiber

> ### MAKES 1 TO 2 SERVINGS

Protein powder makes this smoothie a good option for breakfast. The berries provide a dose of vitamin C, while the flax and chia seeds add omega-3s. For lutein and zeaxanthin, add the optional spinach or kale.

- **Blender**

1 cup	unsweetened coconut milk beverage (approx.)	250 mL
1 cup	frozen berries	250 mL
1 tbsp	flax seeds	15 mL
1 tbsp	chia seeds	15 mL
1	scoop protein powder	1

Optional Add-Ins

¼	avocado, sliced	¼
1 cup	coarsely chopped trimmed spinach or kale	250 mL

1. In blender, combine coconut milk, berries, flax seeds, chia seeds, protein powder and any desired add-ins; blend until smooth. If a thinner consistency is desired, blend in more coconut milk as needed.

Goji Berry Smoothie

EYE NUTRIENTS: Zeaxanthin, vitamin C, vitamin E

Goji berries are an excellent source of zeaxanthin, making this smoothie a carotenoid powerhouse.

TIP: Goji berry powder can be found at health food stores.

• **Blender**

¾ cup	coconut water (approx.)	175 mL
½ cup	raspberries (fresh or frozen)	125 mL
¼ cup	frozen mango chunks	60 mL
¼ cup	sliced peeled cucumber	60 mL
1 tbsp	goji berry powder	15 mL
1 tbsp	coconut oil	15 mL

1. In blender, combine coconut water, raspberries, mango, cucumber, goji berry powder and coconut oil; blend until smooth. If a thinner consistency is desired, blend in more coconut water as needed.

Peach, Pineapple and Pepper Smoothie

EYE NUTRIENTS: Lutein, zeaxanthin, vitamin C

Along with many others in this chapter, this recipe was developed by Dr. Olivia while she was an optometry student and working for Eye Wellness as an intern. She was determined to create a smoothie that included orange peppers and tasted great — mission accomplished! She has since graduated and become an amazing optometrist, and we continue to enjoy her smoothie recipes.

• **Blender**

¾ cup	water (approx.)	175 mL
¼ cup	orange juice	60 mL
¼ tsp	lime juice	1 mL
¼	orange bell pepper, chopped	¼
¾ cup	frozen pineapple chunks	175 mL
¼ cup	frozen sliced peaches	60 mL

1. In blender, combine water, orange juice, lime juice, orange pepper, pineapple and peaches; blend until smooth. If a thinner consistency is desired, blend in more water as needed.

Carrot Mango Smoothie

EYE NUTRIENTS: Beta-carotene, vitamin C, vitamin E

MAKES 1 TO 2 SERVINGS

Here's a great smoothie to serve to kids. They'll love the bright orange color, and they won't even know you've snuck some vegetables in!

- **Blender**

½ cup	unsweetened coconut milk beverage (approx.)	125 mL
¼ cup	orange juice	60 mL
1 tbsp	plain yogurt	15 mL
1 cup	frozen mango chunks	250 mL
¾ to 1 cup	chopped carrots	175 to 250 mL

1. In blender, combine coconut milk, orange juice, yogurt, mango and ¾ cup (175 mL) carrots; blend until smooth. If a thinner consistency is desired, blend in more coconut milk as needed. If a thicker consistency is desired, blend in an additional ¼ cup (60 mL) carrots.

Pumpkin Pie Smoothie

EYE NUTRIENTS: Beta-carotene

MAKES 1 SERVING

This delicious treat tastes more like dessert than a healthy smoothie. It will remind you of pumpkin pie and will definitely satisfy your sweet tooth.

TIP: Make sure to buy pure pumpkin purée and not pumpkin pie filling, which contains added sugar.

- **Blender**

1 cup	unsweetened plain almond milk (approx.)	250 mL
1	frozen banana, broken into chunks	1
½ cup	pumpkin purée (not pie filling)	125 mL
¼ tsp	pumpkin pie spice	1 mL
½ cup	ice cubes	125 mL

1. In blender, combine almond milk, banana, pumpkin, pumpkin pie spice and ice; blend until smooth. If a thinner consistency is desired, blend in more almond milk as needed.

Cantaloupe Drinkable Yogurt

EYE NUTRIENTS: Beta-carotene, vitamin C

MAKES 1 SERVING

Add a dose of beta-carotene and vitamin C to your morning yogurt with cantaloupe cubes. Smoothies don't get easier than this.

- **Blender**

| ½ cup | plain or vanilla-flavored yogurt | 125 mL |
| ¼ | cantaloupe, cut into cubes (about 1 cup/250 mL) | ¼ |

1. In blender, combine yogurt and cantaloupe; blend until smooth.

> **Eyefood Focus**
> Cantaloupe is a source of beta-carotene and vitamin C. For a treat on a hot summer day, freeze cantaloupe chunks and use them in place of ice cubes in a tall glass of sparkling water.

Beta-Carotene Blast

EYE NUTRIENTS: Beta-carotene, vitamin C

MAKES 2 SERVINGS

This juice is a delicious and nutritious way to increase your intake of beta-carotene. The tartness of the grapefruit is a nice contrast to the sweetness of the carrots.

- **Electric juicer**

3	carrots (unpeeled)	3
2	pink grapefruit, peeled and cut into quarters	2
1	lime, peeled	1
	Ice cubes	

1. Following your juicer manual's instructions, juice carrots, grapefruit and lime. Stir together to blend. Serve over ice.

> **Eyefood Focus**
> Beta-carotene is best obtained from food and not supplements. Studies have found that smokers or recent ex-smokers who take a beta-carotene supplement may have an increased risk for lung cancer. However, beta-carotene from food is safe.

Citrus Zinger

EYE NUTRIENTS: Vitamin C

MAKES 2 SERVINGS

This pleasantly tart juice is the ultimate refreshment on a hot, humid day.

TIP: You can use a manual citrus reamer instead of an electric juicer for this recipe. Leave the peels on the fruits and simply cut each piece of fruit in half crosswise to juice.

- **Electric juicer (see tip)**

2	oranges, peeled	2
1	grapefruit, peeled and cut into quarters	1
1	lime, peeled	1
1	lemon, peeled	1
	Fresh mint sprigs (optional)	

1. Following your juicer manual's instructions, juice oranges, grapefruit, lime and lemon. Stir together to blend. Serve immediately, garnished with mint, if desired.

Pear, Ginger and Mint Juice

EYE NUTRIENTS: Lutein, zeaxanthin, vitamin C

MAKES 1 SERVING

Grapefruit adds a pleasing tartness and ginger lends a spicy snap to this nutritious green juice.

- **Electric juicer**

20	fresh mint leaves	20
3	kale leaves, including stem	3
1	pear, chopped	1
1	grapefruit, peeled and cut into quarters	1
1	2-inch (5 cm) piece gingerroot	1
	Ice cubes	

1. Following your juicer manual's instructions, juice mint and kale together, then juice pear, grapefruit and ginger. Stir together to blend. Serve over ice.

Salads
and Dressings

Salads are an integral part of a diet focused on eye health, in part because raw vegetables are an excellent source of vitamin C. Vitamin C is present in every part of the eye, and studies show that eating foods high in antioxidants, including vitamin C, can decrease the risk of cataracts and age-related macular degeneration. Because cooking decreases the amount of vitamin C in foods, salads are a great way to reap the most benefits from veggies.

Salads are also an easy way to include whole grains, beans and lentils in your diet. Feel free to experiment and substitute different whole grains and legumes in these recipes.

Healthy salad dressings are easy to make at home, and they can be made ahead and stored in a jar in your fridge so you can enjoy a salad anytime. Mix and match the dressings in this chapter with any of the salad recipes, or with salads of your own creation!

Create-Your-Own Mason Jar Salad 152

Vegetable Salads

Green Salad with Herbs 153

Mixed Green Salad with Berries
 and Apricots 154

Awesome Arugula Chopped Salad. . . .155

Niçoise Salad 156

Orange Pepper and Kale
 Tossed Salad .157

Mediterranean-Style Kale Salad 158

Mango Spinach Salad 158

Avocado Salad with Radishes 159

Broccoli and Orange Pepper Salad . . . 160

Whole-Grain and Legume Salads

Quinoa and Green Pea Salad. 161

Wheat Berry and Apricot Salad 162

Greek-Style Corn Salad. 163

Kale Salad with Chickpeas 164

Black Bean and Mango Salad 165

Eyefoods Dinner Salad 166

Carrot and Romano Bean Salad 167

Deli-Style Kale Salad. 167

Edamame and Pepper Salad
 with Kalamata Olives. 168

Lentil and Avocado Salad. 168

Lentil and Orange Salad. 169

Chicken and Lentil Salad with Mint. . . .170

Salad Dressings

Basic Salad Dressing. 171

Balsamic Vinaigrette. 171

Citrus Dressing. 172

Creamy Salad Dressing. 172

Creamy Miso Dressing. 173

Orange Curry Dressing. 173

Pumpkin Dressing 174

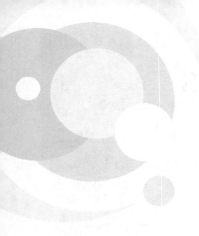

Create-Your-Own Mason Jar Salad

These portable make-ahead salads are a great way to pack wholesome lunches into your week. The key to a crunchy salad is the order of the ingredients. Follow these simple steps to make the perfect mason jar salad. To get your daily dose of lutein and zeaxanthin, choose at least three ingredients with LOL (lots of lutein).

TIP: If you find raw kale too bitter for your palate, give it a rub. Massaging kale leaves causes their tough fibers and cell walls to break down and results in a lighter taste. Massage with olive oil or the dressing called for in the recipe. For an even smoother taste, let stand for 5 minutes, or up to a day, after the rubdown.

1. Make the dressing right in the jar: Add 1 tbsp (15 mL) extra virgin olive oil, 1 tsp (5 mL) apple cider vinegar and ¼ tsp (1 mL) Dijon mustard to the jar and season to taste with salt and freshly ground black pepper. Tighten the lid and shake vigorously until the dressing is mixed.

2. Add grains, a protein and crunchy vegetables:

Grain Suggestions	Protein Suggestions	Crunchy Veggies
Quinoa Wild rice	Hard-cooked egg, chopped (LOL) Cooked turkey breast, sliced Canned light tuna Black beans	Broccoli, chopped (LOL) Carrots, chopped Green peas, frozen (LOL) Orange, red or yellow bell peppers, chopped (LOL) Zucchini, chopped (LOL)

3. Layer on the fixings, such as nuts, seeds and fruit:

Nut Suggestions	Seed Suggestions	Fruit Suggestions
Almonds Walnuts	Chia seeds Green pumpkin seeds (pepitas) Hemp seeds Sunflower seeds	Blueberries, raspberries or sliced strawberries Dried apricots, chopped Dried goji berries

4. Toss in a handful of leafy greens (LOL), such as baby spinach, leaf lettuce, romaine lettuce, watercress, baby kale, radicchio or mixed greens.

5. Cover tightly with a lid and store in the fridge for up to 2 days.

6. To serve, turn the jar upside down onto a plate and dump out the ingredients. Toss together to spread the dressing around, and enjoy your eyefoods!

Green Salad with Herbs

EYE NUTRIENTS: Beta-carotene, lutein, zeaxanthin, vitamin C, vitamin E

This salad features the best green vegetables for eye nutrition. The herbs give it a vibrant and intense flavor. Use local herbs and vegetables for the greatest nutritional benefit.

TIP: After steaming green beans, plunge them into a bowl of ice water to chill, then drain and pat dry. Store them in an airtight container in the fridge to use in salads during the week.

VARIATION: Almost any fresh herbs will work well in this salad. Try mint in place of the dill, and cilantro in place of the parsley.

2 cups	packed torn romaine or leaf lettuce	500 mL
2 cups	packed baby spinach	500 mL
1 cup	bite-size broccoli florets	250 mL
1 cup	sliced green bell pepper	250 mL
1 cup	steamed sliced green beans	250 mL
½ cup	chopped fresh basil	125 mL
½ cup	chopped fresh dill	125 mL
½ cup	chopped fresh parsley	125 mL
3 tbsp	extra virgin olive oil	45 mL
1 tbsp	apple cider vinegar	15 mL
1 tsp	Dijon mustard	5 mL
	Salt and freshly ground black pepper	

1. In a large bowl, toss together lettuce, spinach, broccoli, green pepper, green beans, basil, dill and parsley.

2. In a small bowl, whisk together oil, vinegar and mustard. Season to taste with salt and pepper. Drizzle dressing over salad and toss to coat. Serve immediately.

Mixed Green Salad with Berries and Apricots

EYE NUTRIENTS: Beta-carotene, lutein, zeaxanthin, vitamin C, vitamin E, zinc

Goji berries, apricots and blueberries add a mild sweetness and a pleasant texture to this delicious salad that serves a crowd.

VARIATION: For a sweeter flavor, try a honey Dijon dressing: replace the vinegar with freshly squeezed lemon juice and add 1 tsp (5 mL) liquid honey.

Eyefood Focus

Radicchio, a source of lutein, is native to the Veneto region of northern Italy. Although we include it in the leafy green category, common varieties are actually red and white. Radicchio is harvested in cold weather and has a slightly bitter taste.

1	orange bell pepper, finely chopped	1
1	head leaf or romaine lettuce, torn into bite-size pieces	1
2 cups	packed torn radicchio (bite-size pieces)	500 mL
½ cup	blueberries	125 mL
¼ cup	dried goji berries	60 mL
¼ cup	dried apricots, chopped	60 mL
¼ cup	sunflower seeds	60 mL
3 tbsp	extra virgin olive oil	45 mL
1 tbsp	apple cider vinegar	15 mL
1 tsp	Dijon mustard	5 mL
	Salt and freshly ground black pepper	

1. In a large bowl, toss together orange pepper, lettuce and radicchio. Add blueberries, goji berries, apricots and sunflower seeds.

2. In a small bowl, whisk together oil, vinegar and mustard. Season to taste with salt and pepper. Drizzle dressing over salad and toss to coat. Serve immediately.

Awesome Arugula Chopped Salad

EYE NUTRIENTS: Beta-carotene, lutein, zeaxanthin, vitamin C, vitamin E, omega-3s (DHA and EPA)

MAKES 2 SERVINGS

This chopped salad makes a great meal. The sardines provide protein and are a great source of the omega-3 fatty acids DHA and EPA. If sardines aren't your favorite, you can sub in canned light tuna or salmon.

TIP: As described in this salad, the simple act of chopping can elevate an average salad into a gourmet treat. A mezzaluna would also work well for this task; to use one, chop the ingredients in one direction, then rotate the mezzaluna 90 degrees and chop in the other direction.

1 cup	packed arugula	250 mL
1 cup	packed spinach leaves	250 mL
1	can (3.75 oz/106 g) skinless boneless sardines, drained and chopped	1
6	dill pickle slices	6
2 tbsp	drained capers	30 mL
1 tbsp	prepared mustard	15 mL

1. In a medium bowl, toss together arugula, spinach, sardines and pickles. Using two sharp knives cutting in opposite directions in the bowl, cut into a chopped salad. Add capers and mustard, tossing gently to coat. Serve immediately.

Niçoise Salad

EYE NUTRIENTS: Lutein, vitamin C, vitamin E, omega-3s (DHA and EPA)

MAKES 2 SERVINGS

Here's a twist on the classic niçoise salad, with sardines in place of anchovies or tuna. If you prefer, you can use canned light tuna or grilled fresh or frozen tuna instead.

TIP: To blanch green beans, add them to a pot of boiling water for 2 minutes, then plunge them into a bowl of ice water to chill. Drain and pat dry. Make extras and store them in an airtight container in the fridge to use in salads during the week.

VARIATION: Substitute kale for the spinach or romaine lettuce to make this salad even more of a lutein powerhouse.

Eyefood Focus

To increase your body's absorption of lutein, consume foods that are high in lutein along with foods that contain healthy fats. The green vegetables and eggs, which are high in lutein, combined with the sardines, which are high in omega-3 fatty acids, make this salad a very nutritious meal.

2 cups	packed torn romaine lettuce	500 mL
2 cups	packed baby spinach	500 mL
4	black olives	4
1	green onion, thinly sliced	1
1	hard-cooked egg, cut in half	1
1	can (3.75 oz/106 g) boneless skinless sardines, drained and chopped	1
½ cup	green beans, blanched (see tip)	125 mL
1 tbsp	drained capers, coarsely chopped	15 mL
½ cup	Citrus Dressing (page 172)	125 mL

1. Divide lettuce and spinach between two plates. Arrange olives, green onion, egg, sardines, green beans and capers on top, dividing equally. Drizzle with dressing. Serve immediately.

Orange Pepper and Kale Tossed Salad

MAKES 2 SERVINGS

Green olives add a pleasant tanginess to this dish. If you don't have any on hand, you can substitute capers.

VARIATIONS: Add 1 cup (250 mL) finely chopped red or yellow bell pepper to create "rainbow" salad.

Substitute green pumpkin seeds (pepitas) for the pistachios. Pumpkin seeds are a good source of zinc.

Eyefood Focus

Kale is the highest food source of lutein and is also a great source of vitamin C, vitamin E and beta-carotene. Although we absorb lutein from cooked food better, there is so much lutein in kale that consuming it raw still nourishes us with a high amount of lutein.

2 cups	finely chopped trimmed kale leaves	500 mL
1 cup	finely chopped orange bell pepper	250 mL
¼ cup	sliced pitted green olives	60 mL
1 tbsp	extra virgin olive oil	15 mL
1 tsp	white wine vinegar	5 mL
	Salt and freshly ground black pepper	
¼ cup	chopped pistachios	60 mL

1. In a medium bowl, toss together kale, orange pepper and olives. Add oil and vinegar, tossing to coat. Season to taste with salt and pepper. Cover and refrigerate for at least 1 hour or up to 1 day. Sprinkle with pistachios just before serving.

Mediterranean-Style Kale Salad

EYE NUTRIENTS: Beta-carotene, lutein, zeaxanthin, vitamin C, vitamin E

MAKES 4 SERVINGS

This kale salad is one of the first eyefoods recipes that Dr. Barb and I developed, and it's a lutein and zeaxanthin powerhouse. The sun-dried tomatoes add a nice contrast to the kale.

TIPS: If you prefer your kale more tender, choose bunches that have smaller leaves, as they are younger and will be less fibrous. You can also buy baby kale in boxes.

If you let the kale soak in the dressing overnight, it will have a softer texture.

3½ oz	kale leaves	100 g
4	green onions, thinly sliced	4
1	orange bell pepper, chopped	1
¼ cup	drained oil-packed sun-dried tomatoes, chopped	60 mL
¼ cup	Balsamic Vinaigrette (page 171)	60 mL
¼ cup	toasted pine nuts	60 mL

1. Remove ribs from kale leaves and roughly chop kale into bite-size pieces.

2. In a large bowl, toss together kale, green onions, orange pepper and sun-dried tomatoes. Drizzle with vinaigrette and toss to combine. Cover and refrigerate for at least 1 hour or up to 1 day. Sprinkle with pine nuts just before serving.

Mango Spinach Salad

EYE NUTRIENTS: Lutein, zeaxanthin, vitamin C, vitamin E, zinc

MAKES 4 SERVINGS

Here's a simple salad that is ready in no time and is a great source of vitamin E and lutein.

TIP: Substitute torn radicchio, kale or mixed greens for the baby spinach.

1	mango, sliced	1
4 cups	packed baby spinach	1 L
1 cup	frozen green peas, thawed	250 mL
2 tbsp	green pumpkin seeds (pepitas)	30 mL
2 tbsp	extra virgin olive oil	30 mL
1 tbsp	apple cider vinegar	15 mL
	Salt and freshly ground black pepper	

1. In a large bowl, toss together mango, spinach, peas and pumpkin seeds. Add oil and vinegar, tossing to coat. Season to taste with salt and pepper. Serve immediately.

> **Eyefood Focus**
> Vitamin E is typically found in oils and other fats. For a fruit, though, mango is a good source of vitamin E, making it a great food choice for people following a low-fat diet.

Avocado Salad with Radishes

EYE NUTRIENTS: Lutein, vitamin C, vitamin E, omega-3s (ALA)

You won't be able to get enough of this combination of cucumber, tomato, radish, green onion and avocado. It's a satisfying treat.

Eyefood Focus

Avocado is actually a fruit. It is a source of plant-based omega-3 fatty acids (ALA), vitamin E and zinc, making it a staple source of healthy fats in any plant-based diet.

1	avocado, chopped	1
1	small cucumber, sliced	1
1	tomato, chopped	1
1	green onion, thinly sliced	1
1 cup	thinly sliced radishes	250 mL
2 tbsp	freshly squeezed lemon juice	30 mL
1 tbsp	extra virgin olive oil	15 mL
	Salt and freshly ground black pepper	

1. In a large bowl, combine avocado, cucumber, tomato, green onion and radishes.

2. In a small bowl, combine lemon juice and oil. Season to taste with salt and pepper. Drizzle dressing over salad and toss gently to coat. Serve immediately or cover and refrigerate for up to 2 hours.

Broccoli and Orange Pepper Salad

EYE NUTRIENTS: Beta-carotene, lutein, zeaxanthin, vitamin C, vitamin E

This simple salad takes no time to make. As an added bonus, it can be prepared the night before, making it a great addition to kids' lunch boxes. The carrots and pepper add a nice contrast to the broccoli, in both color and crunch.

VARIATION: Add ¾ cup (175 mL) chopped cooked chicken or turkey breast for a protein punch.

Eyefood Focus

Even though carrots and orange peppers are both orange in color, carrots are known for their high level of beta-carotene, while orange peppers are high in zeaxanthin.

1	orange bell pepper, sliced	1
1	carrot, thinly sliced	1
2 cups	bite-size broccoli florets	500 mL
2 tbsp	extra virgin olive oil	30 mL
1 tbsp	apple cider vinegar	15 mL
1 tbsp	mayonnaise	15 mL
1 tbsp	liquid honey	15 mL
	Salt and freshly ground black pepper	

1. In a medium bowl, combine orange pepper, carrot and broccoli.

2. In a small bowl, whisk together oil, vinegar, mayonnaise and honey. Season to taste with salt and pepper. Drizzle dressing over salad and toss to coat. Cover and refrigerate for at least 1 hour or up to 1 day.

Quinoa and Green Pea Salad

EYE NUTRIENTS: Lutein, zeaxanthin, vitamin C, vitamin E, zinc, fiber

This salad makes a great side to a grilled or poached salmon fillet. If you can find fresh peas, especially in the spring, they make a great substitution for frozen.

VARIATION: Substitute barley or wheat berries for the quinoa.

Eyefood Focus

Quinoa is a complete protein, so it's a great grain choice for people following plant-based diets.

½ cup	oil-packed sun-dried tomatoes	125 mL
1	orange bell pepper, chopped	1
2 cups	frozen green peas, thawed	500 mL
2 cups	cooked quinoa	500 mL
2 tbsp	green pumpkin seeds (pepitas)	30 mL
1 tbsp	freshly squeezed lemon juice	15 mL
1 tsp	Dijon mustard	5 mL
1 tsp	liquid honey	5 mL
	Salt and freshly ground black pepper	

1. Drain sun-dried tomatoes, reserving 3 tbsp (45 mL) oil. Chop tomatoes.

2. In a large bowl, combine chopped tomatoes, orange pepper, peas, quinoa and pumpkin seeds.

3. In a small bowl, whisk together reserved sun-dried tomato oil, lemon juice, mustard and honey. Season to taste with salt and pepper. Drizzle dressing over salad and toss gently to coat. Serve immediately or cover and refrigerate for up to 2 days.

Wheat Berry and Apricot Salad

EYE NUTRIENTS: Beta-carotene, vitamin E, zinc, fiber

MAKES 4 TO 6 SERVINGS

Wheat berries give this salad a pleasant chewy texture. Dried apricots are high in beta-carotene, but when you feel like changing it up, you can substitute dried cranberries.

VARIATION: For a gluten-free option, substitute brown rice for the wheat berries.

¼ cup	oil-packed sun-dried tomatoes	60 mL
10	dried apricots, diced	10
2	green onions, chopped	2
2 cups	cooked wheat berries (see page 178)	500 mL
⅓ cup	chopped nuts (almonds, walnuts or cashews)	75 mL
¼ cup	chopped fresh parsley (or 2 tbsp/30 mL dried)	60 mL
¼ cup	extra virgin olive oil	60 mL
¼ cup	freshly squeezed lemon juice	60 mL
¼ cup	liquid honey	60 mL
	Salt and freshly ground black pepper	

1. Drain sun-dried tomatoes, reserving 2 tbsp (30 mL) oil. Thinly slice tomatoes.

2. In a large bowl, combine sliced tomatoes, apricots, green onions, wheat berries, nuts and parsley.

3. In a small bowl, whisk together reserved sun-dried tomato oil, olive oil, lemon juice and honey. Season to taste with salt and pepper. Drizzle dressing over salad and toss gently to coat. Serve immediately or cover and refrigerate for up to 2 days.

Greek-Style Corn Salad

EYE NUTRIENTS: Lutein, zeaxanthin, vitamin C, vitamin E, zinc, fiber

MAKES 8 TO 10 SERVINGS

This take on Greek salad contains lots of zeaxanthin from the orange pepper and corn. To save time, you can use thawed frozen corn kernels in place of fresh.

TIP: This salad tastes best when served at room temperature, so let it warm up after marinating.

VARIATION: Black beans make a good substitution for the chickpeas and offer a nice color contrast, making the salad visually appealing.

Eyefood Focus

Corn is a source of zeaxanthin, though it doesn't contain as much as orange peppers or goji berries.

4	ears corn, grilled or boiled	4
1	red bell pepper, chopped	1
1	orange bell pepper, chopped	1
1	red onion, chopped	1
1	can (14 to 19 oz/398 to 540 mL) chickpeas, drained and rinsed	1
1	clove garlic, minced	1
2 tbsp	extra virgin olive oil	30 mL
2 tbsp	red wine vinegar	30 mL
	Salt and freshly ground black pepper	
4 oz	feta cheese, crumbled	125 g
	Chopped fresh basil	

1. Using a serrated knife, cut corn kernels off the cob into a medium bowl. Add red pepper, orange pepper, onion and chickpeas.

2. In a small bowl, whisk together garlic, oil and vinegar. Drizzle dressing over salad and toss gently to coat. Cover and refrigerate for at least 2 hours or up to 2 days.

3. Let salad stand at room temperature for about 30 minutes before serving. Season to taste with salt and pepper. Sprinkle with feta and basil just before serving.

Kale Salad with Chickpeas

EYE NUTRIENTS: Beta-carotene, lutein, zeaxanthin, vitamin C, vitamin E, zinc, fiber

Chickpeas add a pleasant chewiness to this salad and are a good source of protein, fiber and zinc.

TIP: You can use roasted red peppers from a jar for this salad. Alternatively, roast your own by cutting peppers in half, removing the seeds and placing peppers cut side down on a foil-lined baking sheet. Broil for about 10 minutes or until the skin is charred. Remove from oven and tent with foil for 15 minutes, then peel off skins.

> **Eyefood Focus**
>
> All peppers are a good source of vitamin C. Orange peppers contain the most, but you can include all of the various colors in your diet for variety.

3½ oz	kale leaves, cut into bite-size pieces	100 g
¼ cup	rinsed drained canned chickpeas	60 mL
¼ cup	drained sliced roasted red bell peppers	60 mL
¼ cup	chopped dried apricots or golden raisins	60 mL
2 tbsp	chopped pitted black olives	30 mL
2 tbsp	mayonnaise	30 mL
2 tbsp	extra virgin olive oil	30 mL
2 tsp	apple cider vinegar, white wine vinegar or unseasoned rice vinegar	10 mL
2 tsp	liquid honey or pure maple syrup	10 mL
	Salt and freshly ground black pepper	

1. In a large bowl, toss together kale, chickpeas, roasted peppers, apricots and olives.

2. In a small bowl, whisk together mayonnaise, oil, vinegar and honey. Season to taste with salt and pepper. Drizzle dressing over salad and toss gently to coat. Cover and refrigerate for at least 1 hour or up to 3 hours.

Black Bean and Mango Salad

EYE NUTRIENTS: Lutein, zeaxanthin, vitamin C, vitamin E, zinc, fiber

MAKES 4 SERVINGS

When I host dinner parties or backyard barbecues, this salad is usually one of my offerings. It can be made the night before, and its vibrant flavors and colors make it a feast for both the taste buds and the eyes.

TIP: If you like heat, you can add more jalapeño pepper. Leaving the seeds in the jalapeño also increases the spiciness. Alternatively, add hot pepper sauce or hot pepper flakes to taste just before serving.

2	green onions, finely chopped	2
1	mango, chopped	1
1	jalapeño pepper, seeded and chopped (optional)	1
1	orange bell pepper, chopped	1
½	red bell pepper, chopped	½
1	can (14 to 19 oz/398 to 540 mL) black beans, drained and rinsed	1
3 tbsp	chopped fresh parsley or cilantro (or 1½ tsp/7 mL dried)	45 mL
	Grated zest of 1 lime	
3 tbsp	extra virgin olive oil	45 mL
2 tbsp	apple cider vinegar	30 mL
1 tbsp	freshly squeezed lime juice	15 mL
1 tsp	Dijon mustard	5 mL
	Salt and freshly ground black pepper	

1. In a large bowl, combine green onions, mango, jalapeño (if using), orange pepper, red pepper, beans, parsley and lime zest.

2. In a small bowl, whisk together oil, vinegar, lime juice and mustard. Season to taste with salt and pepper. Drizzle dressing over salad and toss gently to coat. Cover and refrigerate for at least 1 hour or overnight.

Eyefoods Dinner Salad

EYE NUTRIENTS: Lutein, zeaxanthin, vitamin C, vitamin E, zinc

I enjoy salads for dinner quite often. This one is a staple in my house, as it can easily be changed up with a variety of substitutions. It includes all three macronutrients — carbohydrates, protein and healthy fat — making it a great meal on its own.

VARIATIONS: Substitute torn leaf lettuce or radicchio for the romaine lettuce.

Replace the peas with chopped zucchini or steamed green beans.

Use chopped cashews, walnuts or pistachios in place of the almonds.

Substitute sunflower seeds for the pumpkin seeds.

Use ½ cup (125 mL) chopped mango or cantaloupe in place of the orange.

Replace the black beans with lentils, cannellini (white kidney) beans or chickpeas.

½	orange bell pepper, finely chopped	½
½	orange, chopped	½
1 cup	chopped romaine lettuce	250 mL
1 cup	packed baby spinach	250 mL
½ cup	frozen green peas, thawed	125 mL
½ cup	rinsed drained canned black beans	125 mL
¼ cup	slivered almonds	60 mL
1 tbsp	green pumpkin seeds (pepitas)	15 mL
¼ cup	Orange Curry Dressing (page 173)	60 mL

Protein Additions (Choose 1)

4	hard-cooked eggs, peeled and quartered	4
1½ cups	chopped cooked turkey breast	375 mL
1	can (6 oz/170 g) light tuna or salmon	1

1. In a large bowl, combine orange pepper, orange, romaine, spinach, peas, beans, almonds, pumpkin seeds, and your choice of protein. Drizzle dressing over salad and toss to coat. Serve immediately.

Eyefood Focus

Hard-cooked eggs add an extra burst of lutein and vitamin E to this salad; turkey breast adds more zinc and vitamin E; tuna or salmon contributes omega-3 fatty acids (DHA and EPA).

Carrot and Romano Bean Salad

EYE NUTRIENTS: Beta-carotene, vitamin C, vitamin E, zinc, fiber

MAKES 2 SERVINGS

The crunchiness of carrots makes a nice contrast to the chewiness of the beans in this salad. It's a delicious way to increase your daily intake of fiber.

TIPS: It is not necessary to let the salad marinate, but the flavors will blend and be enhanced as the dressing permeates the vegetables.

Drink lots of water to help reduce the gassy effects of beans.

2	carrots, thinly sliced	2
½	red bell pepper, sliced	½
1 cup	rinsed drained canned Romano beans or cannellini (white kidney) beans	250 mL
2 tbsp	extra virgin olive oil	30 mL
1 tbsp	apple cider vinegar	15 mL
1 tbsp	mayonnaise	15 mL
1 tbsp	pure maple syrup	15 mL
	Salt and freshly ground black pepper	

1. In a medium bowl, combine carrots, red pepper and beans.
2. In a small bowl, whisk together oil, vinegar, mayonnaise and maple syrup. Season to taste with salt and pepper. Drizzle dressing over salad and toss gently to coat. Refrigerate for at least 1 hour or overnight.

Deli-Style Kale Salad

EYE NUTRIENTS: Beta-carotene, lutein, zeaxanthin, vitamin C, vitamin E, zinc, omega-3s (ALA)

MAKES 4 SERVINGS

Here's an eyefoods take on the broccoli salad often seen on the menu in delicatessens. The creamy dressing pairs well with the kale and adds a mild sweetness.

TIP: Roasted soy beans can be found in the snack food aisle at well-stocked supermarkets. They're a good snack when you need a protein boost, and they make a great garnish for salads.

3½ oz	kale leaves	100 g
4	green onions, thinly sliced	4
1	carrot, shredded	1
¼ cup	chopped dried figs or apricots	60 mL
⅓ cup	Creamy Salad Dressing (page 172) or Creamy Miso Dressing (page 173)	75 mL
¼ cup	roasted soy beans (see tip)	60 mL

1. Remove ribs from kale leaves and roughly chop kale into bite-size pieces.
2. In a large bowl, toss together kale, green onions, carrot and figs. Drizzle dressing over salad and toss to coat. Cover and refrigerate for at least 1 hour or up to 3 hours. Sprinkle with soy beans just before serving.

Edamame and Pepper Salad with Kalamata Olives

EYE NUTRIENTS: Lutein, zeaxanthin, vitamin C, vitamin E, omega-3s (ALA), fiber

MAKES 4 SERVINGS

Make this salad the night before and enjoy it for lunch the next day — it gets even tastier as it sits. It also makes a great addition to a summer barbecue.

Eyefood Focus

Parsley is a source of lutein, making it a great addition to an eye-friendly herb garden. Grow parsley in a pot for a tasty addition to salads.

1	orange bell pepper, chopped	1
1	red bell pepper, chopped	1
1 cup	steamed shelled edamame, cooled	250 mL
1 cup	frozen corn, thawed	250 mL
¼ cup	chopped fresh parsley	60 mL
¼ cup	kalamata olives, sliced	60 mL
2 tbsp	extra virgin olive oil	30 mL
1 tbsp	unseasoned rice vinegar	15 mL
	Salt and freshly ground black pepper	

1. In a large bowl, combine orange pepper, red pepper, edamame, corn, parsley and olives. Add oil and vinegar, tossing to coat evenly. Season to taste with salt and pepper. Serve immediately or cover and refrigerate for at least 1 hour or up to 1 day.

Lentil and Avocado Salad

EYE NUTRIENTS: Vitamin C, vitamin E, zinc, omega-3s (ALA), fiber

MAKES 2 SERVINGS

The avocado gives this salad a creamy texture and provides a source of healthy fat. For a high-protein meal, enjoy it as a side to grilled rainbow trout or chicken breast.

VARIATION: Substitute Romano beans for the lentils.

1	avocado, sliced	1
1	red bell pepper, finely chopped	1
¼	red onion, finely chopped	¼
1 cup	cooled cooked lentils or rinsed drained canned lentils	250 mL
1 tbsp	extra virgin olive oil	15 mL
1 tbsp	wine vinegar (either white or red)	15 mL
	Salt and freshly ground black pepper	

1. In a medium bowl, combine avocado, red pepper, onion and lentils. Add oil and vinegar, tossing to coat evenly. Season to taste with salt and pepper. Cover and refrigerate for at least 30 minutes or up to 1 hour.

Lentil and Orange Salad

EYE NUTRIENTS: Vitamin C, vitamin E, zinc, fiber

MAKES 2 SERVINGS

This versatile salad is best made a day ahead to allow the lentils to marinate in the dressing.

TIP: To cook the lentils for this recipe, bring ¾ cup (175 mL) water to a boil. Add just under ½ cup (125 mL) dried green lentils, rinsed well. Return to a boil, then reduce heat to low, cover, leaving lid ajar, and simmer for about 30 minutes or until lentils are tender and water is absorbed.

VARIATIONS: Substitute a mango for the orange, for an extra dash of vitamin E.

Substitute cannellini (white kidney) beans for the lentils.

Eyefood Focus
Lentils are a great low-fat source of protein and should be a staple in any plant-based diet.

	Grated zest of ½ orange	
1	orange, peeled and sliced	1
½	red bell pepper, sliced	½
1 cup	cooled cooked green lentils (see tip) or rinsed drained canned lentils	250 mL
1 to 2 tbsp	chopped fresh mint (or 1 tsp/5 mL dried)	15 to 30 mL
1 tbsp	extra virgin olive oil	15 mL
1 tbsp	freshly squeezed lime juice	15 mL
1 tbsp	apple cider vinegar	15 mL
	Salt and freshly ground black pepper	

1. In a medium bowl, combine orange zest, orange slices, red pepper, lentils and mint to taste.

2. In a small bowl, whisk together oil, lime juice and vinegar. Season to taste with salt and pepper. Drizzle dressing over salad and toss gently to coat. Serve immediately or cover and refrigerate for up to 2 days.

Chicken and Lentil Salad with Mint

EYE NUTRIENTS: Beta-carotene, vitamin E, zinc, fiber

MAKES 1 TO 2 SERVINGS		

I often keep cooked lentils and chicken in the fridge or freezer, enabling me to quickly toss ingredients together for a one-dish meal. But if you have freshly cooked chicken and lentils, this salad tastes great warm too!

VARIATION: Substitute cooked brown rice or barley for the lentils.

Eyefood Focus

Apricots are a source of beta-carotene. Keep in mind that dried apricots have a higher sugar content than fresh, as the sugar becomes concentrated when the fruit is dried.

1 tbsp	extra virgin olive oil	15 mL
1 tbsp	apple cider vinegar	15 mL
1 tbsp	freshly squeezed lime juice	15 mL
10 to 12	fresh mint sprigs	10 to 12
4	dried or fresh chopped apricots	4
1	chicken breast, cooked and sliced	1
1 cup	cooled cooked green lentils (see tip, page 169) or rinsed drained canned lentils	250 mL
	Salt and freshly ground black pepper	

1. In a medium bowl, combine oil, vinegar and lime juice. Add mint to taste, apricots, chicken and lentils; toss to combine. Season to taste with salt and pepper. Serve immediately or cover and refrigerate for up to 2 days.

Basic Salad Dressing

EYE NUTRIENTS: Vitamin C, vitamin E

It's so easy to make your own dressing, and it stores well in the fridge. Adding a whole garlic clove to the jar enhances the flavor of the dressing without overpowering it.

TIP: If you prefer, you can use a blender, or an immersion blender in a tall cup, to make this dressing.

VARIATION: Change up the type of vinegar to suit your tastes. Balsamic vinegar will give the dressing a sweeter flavor, wine vinegar provides a zesty flavor, and rice vinegar is mellower and more balanced.

- $1\frac{1}{2}$- to 2-cup (375 to 500 mL) jar with lid

$\frac{1}{2}$ cup	extra virgin olive oil	125 mL
3 tbsp	water	45 mL
3 tbsp	apple cider vinegar	45 mL
	Grated zest of $\frac{1}{2}$ lemon	
1 tbsp	freshly squeezed lemon juice	15 mL
1 tbsp	Dijon mustard	15 mL
1 tbsp	liquid honey	15 mL
1 tsp	salt	5 mL
1	clove garlic	1

1. In jar, combine oil, water, vinegar, lemon zest, lemon juice, mustard, honey and salt. Place lid on jar and shake well until dressing has a smooth consistency.

2. Add garlic, seal jar and store in the refrigerator for up to 5 days.

Balsamic Vinaigrette

EYE NUTRIENTS: Vitamin E

This versatile dressing tastes great on most salads, whether the main ingredient is leafy greens, beans or a whole grain such as quinoa or rice.

6 tbsp	extra virgin olive oil	90 mL
3 tbsp	balsamic vinegar	45 mL
1 tbsp	liquid honey or pure maple syrup	15 mL
1 tbsp	Dijon mustard	15 mL
	Salt and freshly ground black pepper	

1. In a small bowl, whisk together oil, vinegar, honey and mustard. Season to taste with salt and pepper.

2. Transfer to a jar or squeeze bottle and store in the refrigerator for up to 2 weeks.

Citrus Dressing

EYE NUTRIENTS: Vitamin C, vitamin E

**MAKES ABOUT ½ CUP
(125 ML)**

Lemon juice and orange juice add a pleasant tartness to this dressing, as well as a vitamin C pick-me-up!

¼ cup	extra virgin olive oil	60 mL
2 tbsp	freshly squeezed lemon juice	30 mL
2 tbsp	freshly squeezed orange juice	30 mL
1 tsp	Dijon mustard	5 mL
	Salt and freshly ground black pepper	

1. In a small bowl, whisk together oil, lemon juice, orange juice and mustard. Season to taste with salt and pepper.

2. Transfer to a jar or squeeze bottle and store in the refrigerator for up to 2 weeks.

Creamy Salad Dressing

EYE NUTRIENTS: Vitamin E

**MAKES ABOUT 1 CUP
(250 ML)**

Creamy salad dressings work well with kale and broccoli salads, especially when they are dressed and then allowed to marinate in the fridge for at least 2 hours or overnight.

6 tbsp	mayonnaise	90 mL
6 tbsp	plain yogurt	90 mL
2 tbsp	apple cider vinegar, white wine vinegar or unseasoned rice vinegar	30 mL
2 tbsp	liquid honey or pure maple syrup	30 mL
	Salt and freshly ground black pepper	

1. In a small bowl, whisk together mayonnaise, yogurt, vinegar and honey. Season to taste with salt and pepper.

2. Transfer to a jar or squeeze bottle and store in the refrigerator for up to 2 weeks.

Creamy Miso Dressing

EYE NUTRIENTS: Vitamin C, vitamin E

6 tbsp	mayonnaise	90 mL
1/4 cup	plain yogurt	60 mL
2 tbsp	miso	30 mL
2 tbsp	freshly squeezed orange juice	30 mL
2 tbsp	agave nectar or pure maple syrup	30 mL

MAKES ABOUT 1 CUP (250 ML)

This dressing, inspired by those served in Japanese restaurants, gives salads a zesty flavor.

1. In a small bowl, whisk together mayonnaise, yogurt, miso, orange juice and agave nectar.

2. Transfer to a jar or squeeze bottle and store in the refrigerator for up to 2 weeks.

Orange Curry Dressing

EYE NUTRIENTS: Vitamin C, vitamin E

2	cloves garlic, minced	2
2 tbsp	curry powder	30 mL
1/2 cup	plain Greek yogurt	125 mL
1/2 cup	freshly squeezed orange juice	125 mL
	Salt and freshly ground black pepper	

MAKES ABOUT 1 1/4 CUPS (300 ML)

Try this dressing on a salad composed of leafy greens, whole grains or beans. The combination of orange juice and curry powder adds a nice complexity to the salad.

1. In a small bowl, whisk together garlic, curry powder, yogurt and orange juice. Season to taste with salt and pepper.

2. Transfer to a jar or squeeze bottle and store in the refrigerator for up to 5 days.

Pumpkin Dressing

EYE NUTRIENTS: Beta-carotene, vitamin C, vitamin E

MAKES ABOUT 1¾ CUPS (425 ML)

Pumpkin gives this dressing a creamy texture and a boost of beta-carotene. The maple syrup adds sweetness and is a nice balance to the cider vinegar.

TIP: If you prefer, you can use a blender, or an immersion blender in a tall cup, to make this dressing.

- 2-cup (500 mL) jar with lid

½ cup	extra virgin olive oil	125 mL
½ cup	pumpkin purée (not pie filling)	125 mL
6 tbsp	water	90 mL
3 tbsp	apple cider vinegar	45 mL
1 tbsp	freshly squeezed lemon juice	15 mL
1 tbsp	pure maple syrup	15 mL
1 tbsp	Dijon mustard	15 mL
1 tsp	salt	5 mL
	Freshly ground black pepper	

1. In jar, combine oil, pumpkin, water, vinegar, lemon juice, maple syrup, mustard, salt and pepper to taste. Place lid on jar and shake well until dressing has a smooth consistency.

2. Seal jar and store in the refrigerator for up to 2 weeks.

Starters, Side Dishes and Sauces

Creating a balanced meal involves being creative with your accompaniments. You will be consuming a lot of vegetables when following an eye-friendly diet. Making it a habit to include veggies in your starters, side dishes and sauces will help you reach the recommended daily intakes of eye-healthy nutrients.

The Eyefoods Plan recommends eating both raw and cooked vegetables, as raw veggies are a better source of vitamin C, while cooked veggies are a better source of lutein. You'll get plenty of raw vegetables from the salads in the previous chapter; this one focuses on cooked vegetables.

This chapter begins with some basic guidelines that will allow you to create your own fantastic vegetable side dishes by experimenting with sautéing different types of leafy greens, roasting an array of vegetables and cooking various whole grains. Then, in addition to some side dishes that expand on these themes, I've also provided recipes for terrific starters and sauces to accompany your meals.

Mix-and-Match Sautéed Greens...176
Roasted Veggies 177
Cooking Whole Grains 178

Turkey and Mango Orange Pepper Boats............................179
Broccoli and Spinach Soup 180
Sweet Potato and Orange Pepper Soup...............................181
Sautéed Greens with Sweet Potato and Pear.......................182
Rapini with White Beans and Red Pepper 183
Sautéed Savoy Cabbage...184
Carrot Fries..185
Roasted Butternut Squash and Cauliflower 186
Citrus Mint Salsa...187
Roasted Pepper Coulis 187
Kale Pesto 188

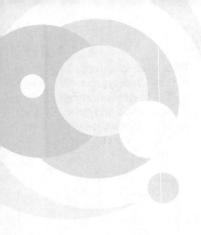

Mix-and-Match Sautéed Greens

It is important to eat a variety of leafy green vegetables, as each type contains a unique ratio of nutrients that are vital for eye health. Try sampling all of the different varieties to give your eyes and body the best health benefits. Enjoying tasty leafy greens is as easy as 1, 2, 3, 4:

1. In a large skillet, sauté 1 clove minced garlic in 1 tbsp (15 mL) olive oil over medium-high heat for 1 minute or until fragrant.

2. Add 8 cups (2 L) leafy greens and 2 tbsp (30 mL) water; stir, then cover, leaving lid ajar, and steam for 30 seconds to 2 minutes or until greens begin to wilt.

3. Add the toppings of your choice to the skillet.

4. Enjoy alone or atop a base, drizzled with balsamic vinegar, rice vinegar or chile-infused olive oil.

Leafy Greens	Toppings	Base
Beet greens Bok choy Collard greens Dandelion greens Escarole Kale Rapini Spinach Turnip or mustard greens	Nuts (slivered almonds, pine nuts, chopped walnuts, ground Eyefoods Nut Mix) Seeds (pumpkin seeds, sesame seeds, sunflower seeds) Thinly sliced bell pepper (orange, red or yellow) Cooked cannellini (white kidney) beans or chickpeas Dry whole wheat bread crumbs Chopped sun-dried tomatoes Slivered gingerroot (sauté with the garlic or add as a topping) Grated lemon zest and juice Chopped dried apricots	Toasted whole-grain baguette Whole wheat pita Toasted corn tortilla Grilled polenta (cornmeal) Baked sweet potato

Tried and True Combinations

- Rapini and 2 tbsp (30 mL) ground Eyefoods Nut Mix (page 222)
- Baby spinach, 4 chopped dried apricots and 3 tbsp (45 mL) pine nuts
- Swiss chard, 2 tbsp (30 mL) ground Eyefoods Nut Mix and 2 tbsp (30 mL) sun-dried tomatoes

Creative Ways to Enjoy Sautéed Greens

- Toast a whole wheat baguette, drizzle with olive oil and top with sautéed greens, for a tasty twist on bruschetta.
- Top a whole wheat pita with olive oil, sautéed greens and shredded mozzarella cheese, for a healthy pizza.
- Slice premade polenta (you can purchase it in logs at the grocery store), place on a rimmed baking sheet and brush with olive oil. Top with sautéed greens and shredded cheese. Bake at 350°F (180°C) until cheese melts.

Roasted Veggies

Once you start roasting vegetables, you will realize how quick and easy it is to add a healthy side dish to your meal. We typically think of roasting root vegetables, such as sweet potatoes and beets, but almost any vegetable will cook nicely on a baking sheet in the oven. Follow these steps to prepare a variety of delicious and nutritious roasted veggies.

Vegetables with a longer cooking time (30–45 minutes)	Vegetables with a shorter cooking time (25–30 minutes)	Seasonings
Beets Brussels sprouts Carrots Parsnips Sweet potatoes Turnips	Asparagus Bell peppers (orange, red or yellow) Broccoli Cauliflower Eggplant Onions Zucchini	Anise seeds Black pepper Chili powder Ground coriander Ground cumin Garlic powder Paprika Salt Ground turmeric

1. Preheat oven to 375°F (190°C) and line a rimmed baking sheet with parchment paper.
2. Choose two or three vegetables (see tip) and cut them into pieces of equal size — about $1\frac{1}{2}$ inches (4 cm) — placing them in a large bowl. Toss with 1 tbsp (15 mL) olive oil for every 2 cups (500 mL) vegetables and the seasonings of your choice until evenly coated.
3. Spread veggies in a single layer on prepared baking sheet and roast for 25 to 45 minutes, depending on the vegetables, until fork-tender. For even browning, turn the vegetables halfway through the cooking time.

TIPS: Adding water to the skillet with the greens prevents burning. You can also simply use freshly washed greens with water still clinging to them.

Eight cups (2 L) of raw leafy greens yields about 1 cup (250 mL) cooked greens, or two servings.

Kale, collard greens and bok choy tend to need a longer steaming time than other greens, closer to 2 minutes.

TIPS: If you choose to mix heartier root vegetables with softer vegetables, chop the heartier vegetables smaller than the softer vegetables so that they will cook in the same time.

Make a large batch of roasted veggies at the beginning of the week and refrigerate them in an airtight container. Prepped and ready to go, they make a great addition to salads and soups.

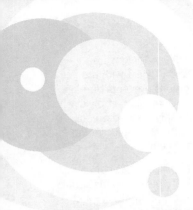

Cooking Whole Grains

The Eyefoods Plan recommends eating ½ cup (125 mL) of cooked whole grains four times a week and enjoying a variety of grains. This chart provides simple instructions on how to prepare some of the healthiest whole grains. I like to pick one or two grains each week and cook enough for the whole family to enjoy over the week. The cooked grains can be stored in an airtight container in the fridge for up to 5 days.

Grain (1 cup/250 mL dry)	Water	Cooking Method	Yield
Barley (hulled)	3 cups (750 mL)	Add barley to boiling water. Reduce heat to low, cover and simmer for 1 hour or until tender. Drain off any remaining water.	3 cups (750 mL)
Barley (pearl)	2 cups (500 mL)	Add barley to boiling water. Reduce heat to low, cover and simmer for 30 to 40 minutes or until tender. Drain off any remaining water.	3½ cups (875 mL)
Brown basmati rice	2 cups (500 mL)	Bring rice and water to a boil. Reduce heat to low, cover and simmer for 35 to 40 minutes or until water is absorbed. Remove from heat and let stand, covered, for 5 minutes, then fluff with a fork.	3 cups (750 mL)
Brown rice (short-, medium- or long-grain)	2 cups (500 mL)	Bring rice and water to a boil. Reduce heat to low, cover and simmer for 40 to 45 minutes or until water is absorbed. Remove from heat and let stand, covered, for 5 minutes, then fluff with a fork.	3 cups (750 mL)
Bulgur (coarse)	2 cups (500 mL)	Bring bulgur and water to a boil. Reduce heat to low, cover and simmer for 12 to 15 minutes or until tender. Drain off any remaining water.	2½ cups (625 mL)
Farro (whole)	3 cups (750 mL)	Add farro to boiling water. Reduce heat to low, cover and simmer for 40 to 60 minutes or until tender. Drain off any remaining water.	2 cups (500 mL)
Quinoa	2 cups (500 mL)	Rinse quinoa well. Add to boiling water. Reduce heat to low, cover and simmer for 15 to 18 minutes or until water is absorbed.	3 cups (750 mL)
Wheat berries	3 cups (750 mL)	Bring water and wheat berries to a boil. Reduce heat to low, cover, leaving lid ajar, and simmer for about 1 hour or until water is absorbed.	2½ cups (625 mL)

Turkey and Mango Orange Pepper Boats

EYE NUTRIENTS: Lutein, zeaxanthin, vitamin C, vitamin E, zinc, omega-3s (ALA)

MAKES 4 TO 8 SERVINGS		

This is one of my favorite appetizers to make when I host a dinner party. It is loved by adults and kids alike and makes a great finger food. Bright and colorful, it is as appealing to your eyes as it is good for them!

TIP: This recipe can be prepared through step 3 up to 1 day ahead and stored in an airtight container in the refrigerator. It can be enjoyed cold or at room temperature.

VARIATION: Replace the turkey with 2 boneless skinless chicken breasts (each about 6 oz/175 g).

Eyefood Focus

Edamame is a source of the plant-based omega-3 fatty acid ALA, making it a good choice for people who do not consume fish.

12 oz	boneless skinless turkey breast, cut into ¼- to ½-inch (0.5 to 1 cm) pieces	375 g
	Salt and freshly ground black pepper	
1 tbsp	olive oil	15 mL
1 cup	frozen shelled edamame	250 mL
2	green onions, chopped	2
1	mango, sliced	1
¼ cup	chopped fresh parsley leaves	60 mL
4	orange bell peppers, cut lengthwise into quarters	4
¼ cup	chopped cashews	60 mL

Dressing

1 tbsp	olive oil	15 mL
1 tbsp	unseasoned rice vinegar	15 mL
1 tsp	reduced-sodium soy sauce	5 mL
1 tsp	freshly squeezed lime juice	5 mL
Dash	hot pepper sauce	Dash
Dash	sesame oil	Dash
	Freshly ground black pepper	

1. Season turkey with salt and pepper. In a large skillet, heat oil over medium-high heat. Add turkey and cook, stirring, for 10 to 12 minutes or until no longer pink inside. Remove from heat.

2. Meanwhile, in a saucepan of boiling water, cook edamame for 2 to 3 minutes or until they float to the top. Drain and rinse under cold water to cool.

3. In a large bowl, combine edamame, green onions, mango and parsley. Add turkey and gently toss to combine.

4. *Dressing:* In a small bowl, whisk together olive oil, vinegar, soy sauce, lime juice, hot pepper sauce, sesame oil and pepper. (Or add all the ingredients to a jar and shake to combine.)

5. Pour dressing over turkey mixture and toss to coat.

6. Arrange orange pepper quarters on a platter. Spoon turkey mixture into peppers and top with cashews.

Broccoli and Spinach Soup

EYE NUTRIENTS: Beta-carotene, lutein, zeaxanthin, vitamin C

MAKES 4 SERVINGS

This healthier version of traditional cream of broccoli soup is a lutein powerhouse, as it includes both broccoli and spinach, each a great source of lutein on its own. The lemon zest and brandy add complexity to the soup's flavor. Serve garnished with sliced toasted almonds or pine nuts.

TIPS: Make sure to use the entire head of broccoli, including the stalks, when making this soup. The stalks may not be as pretty as the florets, but they are filled with nutrients and are just as tasty when puréed.

Using an immersion blender is the easiest way to purée soups. You can use it right in the pot, and cleanup is a breeze.

Eyefood Focus

This recipe will help you meet your weekly targets for both green vegetables (broccoli) and leafy greens (spinach).

- **Blender, food processor or immersion blender**

2 tbsp	olive oil	30 mL
2	stalks celery, chopped	2
2	carrots, chopped	2
$\frac{1}{2}$	large onion, chopped	$\frac{1}{2}$
1	head broccoli, florets and stalks chopped (about $3\frac{1}{2}$ cups/875 mL)	1
2 tbsp	chopped fresh parsley (or 2 tsp/10 mL dried) Grated zest of $\frac{1}{2}$ lemon	30 mL
$\frac{1}{2}$ cup	brandy, white wine or white vermouth	125 mL
4 cups	ready-to-use reduced-sodium chicken broth (approx.)	1 L
1	package (10 oz/284 g) frozen chopped spinach	1
1 cup	milk or unsweetened soy milk	250 mL

1. In a large saucepan, heat oil over medium-high heat. Add celery, carrots and onion; cook, stirring, for 3 to 5 minutes or until onion is translucent. Add broccoli, parsley, lemon zest and brandy; cook, stirring, for 2 minutes.

2. Add broth and bring to a boil. Reduce heat and simmer for 10 to 15 minutes or until broccoli is tender. Add spinach and simmer for 2 to 3 minutes or until spinach is thawed and tender. Remove from heat.

3. In batches as necessary, transfer soup to a blender or food processor and purée until smooth (or use an immersion blender to purée the soup in the pot).

4. Return soup to the pot as needed, place over low heat and stir in milk and, if desired, more broth or water to achieve the desired texture. Cook, stirring, for 2 to 3 minutes or until heated through.

Sweet Potato and Orange Pepper Soup

EYE NUTRIENTS: Beta-carotene, lutein, zeaxanthin, vitamin C

Feast your eyes on this vibrant orange soup that tastes as good as it looks. It makes a great starter for a holiday meal in the autumn or winter.

TIP: For added nutrients, chop baby spinach and place in the bottom of each soup bowl. Add hot soup and let stand for a couple of minutes to soften the spinach before serving.

Eyefood Focus

Watch out, citrus fruit! Half an orange pepper has more than twice as much vitamin C as a medium orange.

- Blender, food processor or immersion blender

2 tbsp	olive oil	30 mL
2	stalks celery, chopped	2
2	carrots, chopped	2
½	large onion, chopped	½
1 lb	sweet potatoes, peeled and chopped	500 g
2	orange bell peppers, chopped	2
1	orange, peeled and chopped	1
2 tbsp	minced gingerroot (or 2 tsp/10 mL ground ginger)	30 mL
¾ cup	dry white wine	175 mL
4 cups	ready-to-use reduced-sodium vegetable or chicken broth (approx.)	1 L

1. In a large saucepan, heat oil over medium-high heat. Add celery, carrots and onion; cook, stirring, for 3 to 5 minutes or until onion is translucent. Add sweet potatoes, orange peppers, orange, ginger and wine; cook, stirring, for 5 minutes.

2. Add broth and bring to a boil. Reduce heat and simmer for 30 to 40 minutes or until sweet potatoes are tender. Remove from heat.

3. In batches as necessary, transfer soup to a blender or food processor and purée until smooth (or use an immersion blender to purée the soup in the pot).

4. Return soup to the pot as needed, place over low heat and, if desired, stir in more broth or water to achieve the desired texture. Cook, stirring, for 2 to 3 minutes or until heated through.

Sautéed Greens with Sweet Potato and Pear

EYE NUTRIENTS: Beta-carotene, lutein, zeaxanthin, vitamin C, vitamin E, zinc, fiber

MAKES 2 SERVINGS

Sweet potato and pear give this side dish a sweet flavor that pairs well with turkey breast. My favorite green for this dish is dandelion greens, but any leafy green will work.

TIPS: Greens will keep in the fridge for anywhere from 3 days to a week. Dandelion greens, arugula and spinach tend to be more delicate and should be consumed within 3 days of purchase; kale, collard greens and rapini have sturdier leaves and will often last up to a week.

The sweet potato can also be cooked in the microwave. Instead of step 1, place the chopped sweet potato in a microwave-safe bowl with 2 tbsp (30 mL) water and microwave on High for 5 minutes or until tender.

- Preheat oven to 375°F (190°C)
- Shallow roasting pan

1	medium sweet potato, peeled and chopped	1
1½ tbsp	olive oil, divided	22 mL
1	Bosc pear, peeled and sliced	1
8 cups	packed spinach leaves, dandelion greens or any other leafy greens	2 L
	Salt and freshly ground black pepper	
	Pure maple syrup or balsamic vinegar	

1. In a small bowl, toss sweet potato with 1½ tsp (7 mL) oil. Spread sweet potato in a single layer on roasting pan. Roast in preheated oven for 30 to 35 minutes or until tender.

2. In a large skillet, heat the remaining oil over medium-high heat. Add pear and cook, stirring often, for 2 to 3 minutes or until softened.

3. Add sweet potato, spinach, and salt and pepper to taste. Cover, leaving lid ajar, and cook for 1 to 2 minutes or until spinach starts to wilt. Uncover and cook, stirring, for 3 to 4 minutes or until spinach is tender but still retains its vibrant color. Remove from heat and drizzle with maple syrup.

Rapini with White Beans and Red Pepper

EYE NUTRIENTS: Beta-carotene, lutein, zeaxanthin, vitamin C, vitamin E, zinc, fiber

MAKES 2 SERVINGS		

Cannellini beans add protein and fiber to this dish, making it a good choice as a hearty accompaniment to a light entrée.

TIPS: Blanching or steaming the rapini before starting step 1 will mellow its flavor. Reduce the cooking time in step 1 to 3 to 5 minutes.

This mixture tastes great as a panini filling — top with cheese, grill and enjoy!

VARIATION: You can substitute any other leafy greens, such as dandelion greens, Swiss chard or beet greens, for the rapini.

2 tbsp	olive oil	30 mL
1	clove garlic, minced	1
½ tsp	hot pepper flakes (optional)	2 mL
8 cups	packed rapini, trimmed and chopped, with water clinging to the leaves	2 L
½	red bell pepper, sliced into long, thin strips	½
1	can (14 to 19 oz/398 to 540 mL) cannellini (white kidney) beans, drained and rinsed	1
	Salt and freshly ground black pepper	
	Additional olive oil or balsamic vinegar (optional)	

1. In a large skillet, heat oil over medium-high heat. Add garlic and hot pepper flakes (if using); cook, stirring, for 1 minute, being careful not to burn the garlic. Add rapini and red pepper; cover, leaving lid ajar, and cook, stirring often, for 5 to 7 minutes or until rapini starts to wilt.

2. Drain off any excess liquid, then stir in beans and season to taste with salt and pepper. Cook, uncovered, for 1 minute. Remove from heat. Drizzle with additional oil or vinegar, if desired.

Sautéed Savoy Cabbage

EYE NUTRIENTS: Beta-carotene, lutein, vitamin C, vitamin E, zinc, fiber

MAKES 4 SERVINGS

Savoy cabbage has a milder, sweeter flavor than red cabbage or other types of leafy greens, so it's a great introduction to this category of vegetable, easing you in before you try greens with a more intense flavor.

TIP: You can use any type of cabbage you prefer in this recipe. Green cabbage is the most common; purple cabbage is sweeter but has tougher leaves. Napa cabbage has an oblong shape and a milder flavor.

Eyefood Focus

While cabbage does not contain as much lutein as other leafy greens, it is a good source of fiber and vitamin C. Add shredded raw cabbage to sandwiches in place of lettuce, or use cabbage leaves in place of tortillas for tacos or wraps.

1 tbsp	olive oil	15 mL
5	slices pancetta (or 4 slices peameal bacon)	5
1	small red onion, chopped	1
1	clove garlic, minced	1
½ tsp	hot pepper flakes	2 mL
½	savoy cabbage	½
2 tbsp	water	30 mL

1. In a large skillet, heat oil over medium-high heat. Add pancetta, onion, garlic and hot pepper flakes; cook, stirring, for 2 to 3 minutes or until onion is translucent.

2. Add cabbage and water; cook, stirring, for 5 to 10 minutes or until cabbage appears translucent and is tender.

Carrot Fries

EYE NUTRIENTS: Beta-carotene, vitamin C, vitamin E, zinc, fiber

MAKES 2 TO 3 SERVINGS

This quick, simple recipe is a great substitute for fries made with white or sweet potatoes. Keep a bag of carrots in your fridge so you can prepare these anytime, and serve them as a side dish or a tasty snack, dipped in a mixture of honey and Dijon mustard.

VARIATIONS: Add 2 tbsp (30 mL) Dijon mustard with the oil in step 1.

Substitute parsnips for some or all of the carrots; they have the same cooking time.

Eyefood Focus

Orange vegetables, including carrots, sweet potatoes and butternut squash, are a great source of beta-carotene, a carotenoid that the body converts to vitamin A. These fries and the roasted squash in the next recipe are both beta-carotene superstars.

- Preheat oven to 400°F (200°C)
- Rimmed baking sheet, lined with parchment paper

4	carrots, cut into 4- by ¼-inch (10 by 0.5 cm) sticks	4
2 tbsp	olive oil	30 mL
1 tsp	chili powder or paprika	5 mL
	Salt and freshly ground black pepper	

1. In a large bowl, combine carrots, oil, chili powder, and salt and pepper to taste, tossing to coat. Spread carrots in a single layer on prepared baking sheet.

2. Roast in preheated oven for 20 to 25 minutes or until tender-crisp.

Roasted Butternut Squash and Cauliflower

EYE NUTRIENTS: Beta-carotene, lutein, vitamin E, fiber

MAKES 6 TO 8 SERVINGS

This roasted veggie dish is a treat in the autumn and winter, when many other fresh vegetables are hard to come by. Serve it with a beef tenderloin roast for an elegant dinner party.

TIP: Make as much of the spice blend as you like, keeping the proportions the same, so you always have some on hand to make this dish. It can be stored in an airtight jar for up to 6 months.

VARIATION: An equal weight of sweet potatoes or carrots can replace the butternut squash.

Eyefood Focus

Cauliflower is a source of the eye nutrients lutein, vitamin C and fiber.

- Preheat oven to 375°F (190°C)
- Rimmed baking sheet, lined with parchment paper

Spice Blend

1 tbsp	paprika	15 mL
1 tsp	ground turmeric	5 mL
1 tsp	ground coriander	5 mL
1 tsp	ground cumin	5 mL
1 tsp	ground cinnamon	5 mL
1 tsp	freshly ground black pepper	5 mL
1/8 tsp	cayenne pepper	0.5 mL
1	butternut squash (about 3 lbs/1.5 kg), diced	1
1	head cauliflower, cut into florets (about 4 cups/1 L)	1
1	bulb fennel, sliced	1
2 tbsp	olive oil	30 mL
	Salt	

1. *Spice Blend:* In a small bowl, combine paprika, turmeric, coriander, cumin, cinnamon, black pepper and cayenne.

2. In a large bowl, combine squash, cauliflower, fennel, oil, spice blend and salt to taste, tossing to coat. Spread vegetables in a single layer on prepared baking sheet.

3. Roast in preheated oven for 30 to 40 minutes or until vegetables are fork-tender.

Citrus Mint Salsa

EYE NUTRIENTS: Vitamin C

**MAKES ABOUT
2 CUPS (500 ML)**

*Serve this salsa with grilled
salmon, rainbow trout,
halibut, chicken or turkey
breast. Or add some canned
black beans and enjoy it as
a salad on its own.*

TIP: The salsa can be stored
in an airtight container in the
refrigerator for up to 2 days.

1	grapefruit, peeled and cut into ¼-inch (0.5 cm) pieces	1
1	small orange, peeled and cut into ¼-inch (0.5 cm) pieces	1
½	bulb fennel, chopped	½
¼ cup	chopped fresh mint	60 mL
	Grated zest and juice of 1 lime	
1 tbsp	olive oil	15 mL
	Salt and freshly ground black pepper	

1. In a small bowl, combine grapefruit, orange, fennel, mint, lime zest, lime juice and oil. Season to taste with salt and pepper.

Roasted Pepper Coulis

EYE NUTRIENTS: Lutein, zeaxanthin, vitamin C, vitamin E, fiber

**MAKES ABOUT
1 CUP (250 ML)**

*A great sauce for eggs
Benedict (see page 129), this
coulis also tastes great with
grilled turkey or chicken
breast, or as a sauce for fish,
gnocchi or pasta. You can
also use it to garnish plates
or creamy soups.*

TIPS: If you don't have garlic-
infused olive oil, use 2 tbsp
(30 mL) regular olive oil and
add ½ clove garlic, coarsely
chopped.

The coulis can be stored in
an airtight container in the
refrigerator for up to 7 days.

- Preheat broiler
- Rimmed baking sheet, lined with foil
- Food processor or blender

1	orange bell pepper	1
1	yellow bell pepper	1
1 tbsp	garlic-infused olive oil (see tip)	15 mL
1 tbsp	olive oil	15 mL
1 tsp	balsamic vinegar or freshly squeezed lemon juice	5 mL
	Salt and freshly ground black pepper	

1. Cut orange and yellow peppers in half and remove stems, seeds and white membranes. Place cut side down on prepared baking sheet. Broil for about 10 minutes or until skins are charred. Remove from oven, tent with foil and let stand for 15 minutes. Remove and discard skins.

2. Transfer peppers to food processor and process until almost smooth. Add garlic-infused oil, olive oil, vinegar, and salt and pepper to taste; process until smooth.

Kale Pesto

EYE NUTRIENTS: Beta-carotene, lutein, zeaxanthin, vitamin C, vitamin E, zinc, fiber

MAKES ABOUT 2 CUPS (500 ML)

My version of pesto adds kale to the traditional basil and pine nuts, making it a great source of lutein, zeaxanthin and vitamin C. Enjoy it tossed with whole wheat pasta or spread over a grilled turkey or chicken breast.

TIPS: The pesto can be stored in an airtight container in the refrigerator for up to 4 days.

If you grow kale and basil in your garden, you can make this in large batches. Freeze the pesto in ice cube trays, then transfer the cubes to freezer bags. Each cube will be about 2 tbsp (30 mL).

VARIATION: Substitute walnuts for the pine nuts to add omega-3s (ALA) and for an earthier taste.

- Food processor

4	cloves garlic, minced	4
4 cups	packed kale (about 3½ oz/100 g), cut into bite-size pieces (you can include the stems)	1 L
½ cup	packed basil leaves	125 mL
½ cup	pine nuts	125 mL
	Juice of ½ lemon	
¼ cup	olive oil	60 mL

1. In food processor, combine garlic, kale, basil, pine nuts and lemon juice; process until well blended. With the motor running, through the feed tube, gradually add oil and blend to a paste-like consistency.

Main Courses

This chapter contains mouthwatering mains that are easy to prepare and full of eye nutrients. You'll see a common theme, with many of the recipes including leafy greens, bell peppers, peas and broccoli for their lutein and zeaxanthin content.

Comforting, hearty and delicious soups and stews lead into the chapter. You can add kale or spinach to almost any soup or stew and create a dish that will nourish your eyes. I often make a large batch and freeze individual servings so I always have a healthy lunch option ready to go.

Filling out the chapter is a wide variety of recipes featuring whole grains, turkey, lean beef and cold-water fish, with some options that are perfect for Meatless Monday.

Soups and Stews

Kale and White Bean Soup 190

Lentil Soup. 191

Kale Soup with Turkey and
Wild Rice 192

Sweet Potato and Lentil Stew 193

Turkey and Orange Pepper Chili
with Lime. 194

Vegetarian Mains

Whole Wheat Penne with Spinach. . . 195

Pasta with Rapini. 196

Broccoli, Edamame and Nut
Rice Bowls 197

Sweet Potato and Kale Bake 198

Crustless Quiche 199

Fish and Seafood

Poached Salmon 200

Crusted Salmon Fillets 201

Mango Tango Salmon. 202

Rainbow Trout Packets. 203

Orecchiette with Baby Peas
and Crab. 204

Grilled Scallop and Pineapple
Skewers 205

Shrimp Stir-Fry. 206

Chicken, Turkey and Beef

Chicken Cacciatore 208

Chicken and Almond
Lettuce Wraps. 209

Chicken and Black Bean Rice Bowls
with Wasabi Lime Sauce. 210

Turkey Stir-Fry with Peanut Sauce . . . 211

Turkey Fajitas 212

Turkey, Pea and Carrot
Barley Bowls 213

Eyefoods Shepherd's Pie 214

Turkey Burgers with Roasted
Orange Peppers 215

Turkey Meatballs in Tomato Sauce . . . 216

Stuffed Orange Peppers. 217

Mom's Eye-Friendly Meatloaf 218

Beef and Broccoli with Barley 219

Mango and Beef Stir-Fry. 220

Kale and White Bean Soup

EYE NUTRIENTS: Beta-carotene, lutein, zeaxanthin, vitamin E, zinc

In addition to being full of eye-healthy nutrients, this hearty vegetarian soup provides protein thanks to the white beans. Enjoy the soup as it is or, for a creamier version, use an immersion blender to gently blend the ingredients at the end.

TIPS: If you have a 28-oz (796 mL) can of pumpkin purée, use half the can and save the other half for another use.

Leftover soup can be stored in airtight containers in the refrigerator for up to 3 days or in the freezer for up to 6 months.

Eyefood Focus

Kale is a member of the Brassica family, which also includes cabbage, Brussels sprouts, turnips, watercress, horseradish and wasabi.

2 tbsp	olive oil	30 mL
2	carrots, chopped	2
2	stalks celery, chopped	2
½	large onion, chopped	½
½ cup	dry white wine	125 mL
4	sprigs fresh tarragon (or 2 tsp/10 mL dried tarragon)	4
1	can (14 to 19 oz/398 to 540 mL) cannellini (white kidney) beans	1
6 cups	ready-to-use chicken broth	1.5 L
1⅔ cups	pumpkin purée (not pie filling)	400 mL
4 cups	chopped trimmed kale	1 L
⅓ cup	brown basmati rice	75 mL

1. In a large pot, heat oil over medium-high heat. Add carrots, celery and onion; cook, stirring, for 4 to 5 minutes or until softened. Add wine and tarragon; cook, scraping up any browned bits from the bottom of the pot, for 2 minutes.

2. Add beans, broth and pumpkin; bring to a boil. Stir in kale and rice; reduce heat and simmer for 35 to 40 minutes or until rice is tender.

Lentil Soup

EYE NUTRIENTS: Lutein, vitamin E, zinc, fiber

MAKES 4 TO 6 SERVINGS

This nourishing soup is satisfying enough to be a meal in its own right. Enjoy it with a slice of whole-grain toast drizzled with olive oil.

TIPS: For a creamier version, gently blend the soup with an immersion blender. You don't need to purée the soup completely, but gently blending it melds the ingredients together in a pleasant way.

Leftover soup can be stored in airtight containers in the refrigerator for up to 4 days or in the freezer for up to 6 months.

2 tbsp	olive oil	30 mL
1	small to medium onion, chopped	1
1	clove garlic, minced	1
½ tsp	dry mustard	2 mL
½ tsp	coriander seeds	2 mL
½ tsp	ground cumin	2 mL
½ tsp	ground turmeric	2 mL
2	carrots, chopped	2
2	stalks celery, chopped	2
½ cup	dry white wine	125 mL
1	can (28 oz/796 mL) diced tomatoes, with juice	1
4 cups	ready-to-use vegetable or chicken broth	1 L
½ cup	pumpkin purée (not pie filling)	125 mL
½ cup	dried red lentils, rinsed	125 mL
½ cup	dried green lentils, rinsed	125 mL
	Freshly ground black pepper	
1 cup	frozen chopped spinach (3½ oz/100 g or 6 cubes), thawed and excess liquid squeezed out	250 mL
	Cayenne pepper	

1. In a medium pot, heat oil over medium-high heat. Add onion, garlic, mustard, coriander seeds, cumin and turmeric; cook, stirring, for about 1 minute or until spices are toasted. Add carrots and celery; cook, stirring, for 4 to 5 minutes or until vegetables are starting to soften. Stir in wine, scraping up any browned bits from the bottom of the pot.

2. Stir in tomatoes, broth and pumpkin; bring to a boil. Stir in red lentils, green lentils and black pepper to taste; reduce heat to medium-low, cover, leaving lid ajar, and simmer, stirring occasionally, for 20 to 25 minutes or until lentils are tender.

3. Stir in spinach and cayenne to taste; simmer, uncovered, for 5 minutes.

Kale Soup with Turkey and Wild Rice

EYE NUTRIENTS: Lutein, zeaxanthin, vitamin E, zinc

MAKES 10 SERVINGS

This soup will keep you warm on a cold winter evening and nourish your eyes. If you save leftover turkey, you can make your own stock, which will save you time and will be much more flavorful than store-bought chicken broth.

TIPS: If you use unsalted turkey stock, add 1 to 2 tsp (5 to 10 mL) salt, to taste, with the stock.

To make cooking easier, prepare and measure all of your ingredients before you start to cook.

Leftover soup can be stored in airtight containers in the refrigerator for up to 3 days or in the freezer for up to 4 months.

Eyefood Focus

Wild rice is actually not a rice but a species of grass. It does not contain gluten and is a good source of fiber, protein and zinc.

2 tbsp	olive oil	30 mL
½ cup	finely sliced green onions	125 mL
¼ cup	wild rice	60 mL
2 tbsp	chopped fresh parsley	30 mL
2 tbsp	chopped fresh chives	30 mL
8 cups	ready-to-use chicken broth or turkey stock	2 L
4 cups	finely chopped trimmed kale	1 L
2 cups	chopped cooked turkey breast	500 mL
	Freshly grated Parmesan cheese	

1. In a large pot, heat oil over medium heat. Add green onions, wild rice, parsley and chives; cook, stirring often, for 2 minutes or until green onions are softened.

2. Stir in broth and bring to a boil over high heat. Reduce heat to medium-low, cover and simmer for 45 minutes or until wild rice is tender.

3. Add kale and turkey; simmer, uncovered, for 5 minutes or until turkey is heated through. Serve garnished with cheese.

Sweet Potato and Lentil Stew

EYE NUTRIENTS: Beta-carotene, lutein, zeaxanthin, vitamin C, vitamin E, zinc, fiber

The spices in this stew give it an Asian twist. If you don't have cumin and turmeric on hand, you can use Mediterranean herbs, such as dried rosemary, thyme and bay leaf, instead.

Eyefood Focus

Lentils are low in fat and calories, but are a great source of protein and fiber. In fact, ½ cup (125 mL) cooked lentils contains about 30% of the eyefoods daily target for fiber.

2 tbsp	olive oil	30 mL
1	clove garlic, minced	1
½	large onion (or 1 small), chopped	½
2 tsp	ground cumin	10 mL
1 tsp	dry mustard	5 mL
½ tsp	ground turmeric	2 mL
Pinch	cayenne pepper (optional)	Pinch
	Water or ready-to-use vegetable broth	
1	carrot, chopped	1
1	sweet potato, peeled and chopped	1
1	red bell pepper, chopped	1
1	orange bell pepper, chopped	1
1	can (28 oz/796 mL) diced tomatoes, with juice	1
½ cup	dry white wine or unsweetened apple juice	125 mL
½ cup	ready-to-use vegetable broth	125 mL
½ cup	pumpkin purée (not pie filling)	125 mL
½ cup	dried red lentils, rinsed	125 mL
1 cup	frozen chopped spinach (3½ oz/100 g or 6 cubes), thawed and excess liquid squeezed out	250 mL
	Salt and freshly ground black pepper	

1. In a large saucepan, heat oil over medium-high heat. Add garlic and onion; cook, stirring, for 2 to 3 minutes or until onions are translucent. Stir in cumin, mustard, turmeric, cayenne (if using) and a little bit of water as needed; cook, stirring, for 1 minute.

2. Stir in carrot, sweet potato, red pepper, orange pepper, tomatoes, wine, broth and pumpkin; bring to a boil. Add lentils, reduce heat to medium-low, cover, leaving lid ajar, and simmer, stirring occasionally, for 45 to 60 minutes or until vegetables are tender.

3. Stir in spinach and simmer, stirring occasionally, for about 2 minutes or until spinach is heated through. Season to taste with salt and pepper.

Turkey and Orange Pepper Chili with Lime

EYE NUTRIENTS: Lutein, zeaxanthin, vitamin C, vitamin E, zinc, fiber

Whether you're throwing a party or looking for a deliciously different make-ahead meal for your family, this zesty chili will feed a crowd or stock your freezer, and is sure to be a hit all year round. It is best prepared at least a day ahead, to allow the flavors to develop.

TIPS: Set out bowls of cubed avocado and chopped fresh cilantro at the table for diners to use as garnish.

Leftover chili can be stored in airtight containers in the refrigerator for up to 3 days or in the freezer for up to 3 months.

Eyefood Focus

Turkey is a great source of zinc, an important nutrient for ocular health. Zinc is necessary for our bodies to transport vitamins A and E from the liver to our retina.

4 tbsp	olive or grapeseed oil (approx.), divided	60 mL
4 lbs	ground turkey	2 kg
3	medium onions, finely chopped	3
6 tbsp	chili powder	90 mL
¼ cup	unsweetened cocoa powder	60 mL
	Salt and freshly ground black pepper	
4	orange bell peppers, finely chopped	4
2	cans (each 28 oz/796 mL) diced tomatoes, with juice	2
2	cans (each 14 to 19 oz/398 to 540 mL) red kidney beans, drained and rinsed	2
	Grated zest and juice of 3 limes	

1. In a large pot, heat 1 tbsp (15 mL) oil over medium-high heat. Working in small batches, add turkey and cook, breaking it up with a spoon, until no longer pink. Using a slotted spoon, transfer turkey to a bowl as it browns and repeat with the remaining turkey, adding more oil and adjusting the heat as needed between batches.

2. Add 2 tbsp (30 mL) oil and onions to the pot and cook, stirring, for about 7 minutes or until onions are softened.

3. Return turkey and any accumulated juices to the pot, stirring well. Add chili powder, cocoa, and salt and pepper to taste; cook, stirring, for 2 to 3 minutes to blend the flavors.

4. Stir in orange peppers and tomatoes; bring to a boil. Reduce heat to medium-low, cover and simmer, stirring occasionally, for 30 minutes.

5. Add beans and simmer, uncovered, stirring occasionally for 30 minutes or until chili has a nice thick consistency. Remove from heat and stir in lime zest and juice.

Whole Wheat Penne with Spinach

EYE NUTRIENTS: Beta-carotene, lutein, zeaxanthin, vitamin C, vitamin E, fiber

MAKES 2 SERVINGS

This pasta dish is quick to prepare and makes a great weeknight dinner. Cooking the spinach in the pasta water makes it a one-pot meal and saves on dishes.

VARIATIONS: For a gluten-free version, substitute buckwheat pasta, chickpea pasta or quinoa pasta. These alternatives are commonly found in the supermarket.

Substitute fresh broccoli florets for the frozen spinach.

2 cups	dried whole wheat penne pasta	500 mL
1½ cups	frozen chopped spinach (5 oz/150 g or 9 cubes)	375 mL
2 tbsp	freshly grated Parmesan cheese	30 mL
2 tbsp	extra virgin olive oil	30 mL
	Salt and freshly ground black pepper	

1. In a medium pot of boiling salted water, cook penne for 8 minutes. Add frozen spinach and cook for about 2 minutes or until pasta is al dente and spinach is heated through. Drain.

2. Transfer penne and spinach to a bowl and toss with cheese and oil. Season to taste with salt and pepper. Serve immediately.

Pasta with Rapini

EYE NUTRIENTS: Beta-carotene, lutein, zeaxanthin, vitamin C, vitamin E, fiber

This dish is a staple in my household. It's quick, tasty and loaded with nutrients.

TIP: Rapini is also called broccoli rabe. To preserve rapini's vibrant color, be sure not to overcook it.

VARIATIONS: Dandelion greens make a great substitute for the rapini.

If you don't follow a vegetarian diet, you can add sautéed sliced turkey sausage or browned ground turkey to increase the protein content of this dish.

	Water	
4 cups	dried whole wheat penne pasta	1 L
4 tbsp	extra virgin olive oil, divided	60 mL
1	clove garlic, minced (or 1 tsp/5 mL garlic powder)	1
¼ tsp	hot pepper flakes	1 mL
14 oz	rapini, trimmed	400 g
¼ cup	sliced black olives	60 mL
	Salt and freshly ground black pepper	
	Freshly grated Parmesan cheese	

1. In a large pot of boiling salted water, cook penne for about 10 minutes or until al dente.

2. Meanwhile, in a skillet, heat 2 tbsp (30 mL) olive oil over medium heat. Add garlic and hot pepper flakes; cook, stirring, for 1 minute or until fragrant. Add rapini and 2 tbsp (30 mL) water; cover and steam for 2 minutes or until rapini is wilted. Add olives and salt and pepper to taste; cook, stirring, for 3 minutes.

3. Drain pasta and add to rapini mixture. Add the remaining oil and toss to coat. Serve immediately, sprinkled with cheese.

Broccoli, Edamame and Nut Rice Bowls

EYE NUTRIENTS: Lutein, zeaxanthin, vitamin C, vitamin E, zinc, omega-3s (ALA), fiber

MAKES 6 SERVINGS

This gluten-free dish makes enough for a crowd and can be enjoyed hot or cold. For a cold salad version, store it in the refrigerator overnight and enjoy it the next day. It makes a great vegetarian meal, but you can add cooked turkey or chicken breast for a boost of protein.

TIP: You can prepare broccoli ahead of time by blanching it: add it to boiling water, cook for about 3 minutes, then plunge it into cold water to stop the cooking process. Store it in the fridge for an easy addition to weeknight meals. Blanching broccoli helps it retain its bright green color.

VARIATION: Substitute quinoa or wild rice for the brown rice, adjusting the cooking time as necessary.

- **Steamer basket**

1 cup	medium-grain brown rice, rinsed	250 mL
	Water	
1	head broccoli, cut into florets	1
3½ cups	frozen shelled edamame	875 mL
¼ cup	unsalted cashews	60 mL
¼ cup	walnut halves	60 mL
2 tbsp	soy sauce, divided	30 mL
1 tsp	cornstarch	5 mL
½ cup	ready-to-use chicken broth	125 mL
	Juice of ½ lime	
1 tbsp	olive oil	15 mL
1 tbsp	grated gingerroot	15 mL

1. In a medium saucepan, bring rice and 2 cups (500 mL) water to a boil over high heat. Reduce heat to low, cover and simmer for 40 to 45 minutes or until water is absorbed. Remove from heat and let stand, covered, for 5 minutes, then fluff with a fork. Keep warm.

2. Meanwhile, in a steamer basket set over a pot of boiling water, steam broccoli and edamame for about 3 minutes or until tender-crisp. Set aside.

3. Heat a small dry skillet over medium-low heat. Add cashews and walnuts; toast, shaking the pan constantly, until nuts are light brown. Remove from heat and stir in 1 tbsp (15 mL) soy sauce. Set aside.

4. In a small bowl, combine cornstarch, broth, lime juice and the remaining soy sauce, stirring until cornstarch is dissolved. Set aside.

5. In a medium skillet, heat oil over medium heat. Add ginger and cook, stirring, for 30 seconds. Add broccoli and edamame; cook, stirring, for 1 minute. Add sauce and cook, stirring, for about 20 seconds or until heated through and thickened.

6. Divide rice among bowls and spoon broccoli mixture over top. Top with nut mixture.

Sweet Potato and Kale Bake

EYE NUTRIENTS: Beta-carotene, lutein, zeaxanthin, vitamin C, vitamin E, fiber

This recipe is a healthy alternative to lasagna, and it can be assembled ahead of time and baked when needed.

TIP: This dish can be assembled through step 3, then wrapped tightly with plastic wrap and stored in the refrigerator for up to 2 days.

Eyefood Focus

Sweet potatoes are the highest food source of beta-carotene, which the body converts into vitamin A. Vitamin A is used by the rods and cones in the retina to create the visual signal.

- **Preheat oven to 375°F (190°C)**
- **13- by 9-inch (33 by 23 cm) glass baking dish**

3 tbsp	water	45 mL
2 cups	trimmed kale leaves	500 mL
1 tbsp	olive oil	15 mL
1	clove garlic, minced (or 1 tsp/5 mL garlic powder)	1
½	medium onion, finely chopped	½
13	fresh sage leaves, chopped	13
1 cup	ricotta cheese	250 mL
	Salt and freshly ground black pepper	
1¾ cups	tomato sauce	425 mL
3 or 4	medium sweet potatoes (about 28 oz/850 g total), peeled and cut lengthwise into ¼-inch (0.5 cm) thick slices	3 or 4
½ cup	shredded mozzarella or freshly grated Parmesan cheese	125 mL

1. In a skillet, bring water to a simmer over high heat. Add kale, cover and steam for about 5 minutes or until kale is tender but still vibrant in color. Drain kale and let cool slightly.

2. Meanwhile, add oil to the skillet and heat over medium heat. Add garlic and onion; cook, stirring, for 2 to 3 minutes or until onion is translucent.

3. Squeeze out excess water from kale, chop and place in a medium bowl. Add onion mixture, sage and ricotta. Season to taste with salt and pepper.

4. Spread ¾ cup (175 mL) tomato sauce over bottom of baking dish. Arrange half the sweet potato slices on top and season lightly with salt and pepper. Spread ricotta mixture over sweet potatoes, then sprinkle with half the mozzarella. Spread ¼ cup (60 mL) tomato sauce on top. Finish with another layer of sweet potatoes, seasoned with salt and pepper, and the remaining tomato sauce and mozzarella. Cover with foil.

5. Bake in preheated oven for 45 to 60 minutes or until sweet potatoes are fork-tender. Uncover and let cool for 15 minutes before serving.

Crustless Quiche

EYE NUTRIENTS: Lutein, zeaxanthin, vitamin C, vitamin E, zinc

Eggs aren't only for breakfast! This meatless main is a healthy way to enjoy quiche, as it eliminates the need for a pastry shell. It can be prepared ahead of time and enjoyed cold for lunch or dinner, with a mixed green salad.

TIP: To make this quiche ahead, prepare it through step 3, let cool completely, then cover with plastic wrap and store in the refrigerator for up to 3 days.

VARIATIONS: In place of the green onions, peppers and kale, try using 2 cups (500 mL) broccoli, ½ cup (125 mL) sun-dried tomatoes and ½ cup (125 mL) sliced kalamata olives.

Use feta cheese in place of Cheddar.

- **Preheat oven to 375°F (190°C)**
- **8-inch (20 cm) square baking dish, greased**

1 tbsp	olive oil	15 mL
2	green onions, chopped	2
1	red or orange bell pepper, chopped	1
3 cups	chopped trimmed kale (bite-size pieces)	750 mL
½ cup	shredded Cheddar cheese	125 mL
6	large omega-3 eggs	6
½ cup	milk	125 mL
	Salt and freshly ground black pepper	
1 tbsp	chopped fresh parsley (or 1 tsp/5 mL dried)	15 mL
1 tbsp	chopped fresh tarragon (or 1 tsp/5 mL dried)	15 mL

1. In a large skillet, heat oil over medium-high heat. Add green onions, red pepper and kale; cook, stirring, for 3 to 5 minutes or until pepper has softened. Transfer to prepared baking dish and sprinkle with cheese.

2. In a large bowl, whisk together eggs and milk. Season with salt and pepper, then stir in parsley and tarragon. Pour over vegetable mixture and stir gently to evenly distribute ingredients.

3. Bake in preheated oven for 18 to 25 minutes or until quiche is set.

Poached Salmon

EYE NUTRIENTS: Omega-3s (DHA and EPA)

Poaching is a healthy way to prepare salmon. Here, the dill, cilantro and fennel in the poaching liquid add a pleasantly tangy flavor. Enjoy hot or cold.

TIP: Enjoy leftover salmon for lunch the next day in a salad of romaine lettuce or spinach.

Eyefood Focus

Salmon is one of the few foods that is naturally high in vitamin D, more commonly obtained from the sun.

2	green onions, coarsely chopped	2
½	lemon, sliced	½
¼	bulb fennel	¼
½ cup	packed fresh dill	125 mL
½ cup	packed fresh cilantro	125 mL
2 tsp	black peppercorns	10 mL
1 tsp	salt	5 mL
8 cups	water	2 L
½ cup	dry white wine	125 mL
20 oz	skinless salmon fillet, cut into 4 pieces	600 g

1. In a medium saucepan, combine green onions, lemon, fennel, dill, cilantro, peppercorns, salt, water and wine. Bring to a simmer over medium-low heat. Reduce heat to low and simmer for 30 minutes. Using a slotted spoon, remove and discard solids.

2. Return liquid to a simmer, add salmon and simmer for 7 to 10 minutes or until fish is opaque and flakes easily when tested with a fork.

Crusted Salmon Fillets

EYE NUTRIENTS: Vitamin E, zinc, omega-3s (DHA and EPA), fiber

MAKES 4 SERVINGS

In this healthy version of breaded fish fillets, the wheat germ, oat bran and almonds are good sources of vitamin E, zinc and fiber. Serve each fillet on a bed of green lentils, with steamed asparagus on the side.

Eyefood Focus

Cold-water fish provides more of the omega-3 fatty acids DHA and EPA than any other food. Other foods, such as eggs, can be enriched with DHA, but you would have to eat 15 eggs to get the same amount of omega-3s as in a 3½-oz (100 mL) salmon fillet.

- Preheat oven to 400°F (200°C)
- Rimmed baking sheet, lined with foil

2 tbsp	wheat germ	30 mL
2 tbsp	oat bran	30 mL
2 tbsp	ground almonds	30 mL
	Salt and freshly ground black pepper	
2 tbsp	Dijon mustard	30 mL
1 tbsp	pure maple syrup	15 mL
1 tbsp	freshly squeezed lemon juice	15 mL
20 oz	skinless salmon fillet, cut into 4 pieces	600 g

1. In a small bowl, combine wheat germ, oat bran, almonds, and salt and pepper to taste.

2. In another small bowl, combine mustard, maple syrup and lemon juice, stirring well.

3. Arrange salmon on prepared baking sheet. Coat tops of salmon with mustard mixture, then sprinkle with wheat germ mixture, pressing to adhere and coat evenly.

4. Bake in preheated oven for 15 to 20 minutes or until fish is opaque and flakes easily when tested with a fork.

Mango Tango Salmon

EYE NUTRIENTS: Lutein, zeaxanthin, vitamin C, vitamin E, omega-3s (DHA and EPA)

Mango salsa gives this dish a tropical flare. I love eating fish with a fruit salsa. Serve brown rice and a green salad on the side.

VARIATIONS: Substitute rainbow trout for the salmon and bake for 10 to 12 minutes.

Peach, pineapple or orange chunks can be used in place of mango.

Eyefood Focus

Salmon contains omega-3s, which keep your eyes healthy by reducing symptoms of dry eye. They may also protect the retina from age-related macular degeneration and help your body absorb lutein and zeaxanthin.

- Preheat oven to 400°F (200°C)
- Rimmed baking sheet, lined with foil

20 oz	skinless salmon fillet, cut into 4 pieces	600 g
1 tbsp	olive oil	15 mL
	Salt and freshly ground black pepper	

Mango Salsa

1	green onion, finely chopped	1
½	orange bell pepper, cut into ¼-inch (0.5 cm) pieces	½
1 cup	fresh or thawed frozen mango chunks, cut into ¼-inch (0.5 cm) pieces	250 mL
1 cup	grape tomatoes, cut into ¼-inch (0.5 cm) pieces	250 mL
	Grated zest and juice of 1 lime	
1 tbsp	olive oil	15 mL
	Salt and freshly ground black pepper	

1. Arrange salmon on prepared baking sheet, brush with oil and sprinkle with a little salt and pepper. Bake in preheated oven for 15 to 20 minutes or until fish is opaque, browned on top and flakes easily when tested with a fork.

2. *Salsa:* Meanwhile, in a medium bowl, gently combine green onion, orange pepper, mango, tomatoes, lime zest, lime juice and oil. Season with a little salt and pepper.

3. Serve salmon topped with salsa.

Rainbow Trout Packets

EYE NUTRIENTS: Lutein, zeaxanthin, vitamin C, vitamin E, zinc, omega-3s (DHA and EPA)

MAKES 4 SERVINGS

My favorite way to prepare fish is to cook it in packets. They're quick to put together, and cleanup is a breeze. I've used rainbow trout in this recipe, but salmon and halibut also work well.

TIPS: Open the packets carefully to avoid getting scalded by the steam that bursts out.

You can prepare the packets through step 2, wrap them well with foil or place them in a freezer bag or airtight container, and freeze for up to 3 months. Cook from frozen, adding 5 to 10 minutes to the cooking time.

- Preheat oven to 350°F (180°C)
- 4 rectangles parchment paper or foil large enough to wrap around a piece of fish
- Large baking sheet

4 cups	chopped trimmed kale	1 L
1	onion, thinly sliced	1
20 oz	rainbow trout fillets, cut into 4 pieces	600 g
½ cup	chopped fresh cilantro or parsley	125 mL
¼ cup	freshly squeezed lemon juice	60 mL
1 tbsp	olive oil	15 mL
	Salt and freshly ground black pepper	
2	small oranges, thinly sliced, including peel	2
2	limes, thinly sliced, including peel	2

1. Create a bed of 1 cup (250 mL) kale in the center of each piece of parchment paper. Top with onion, dividing evenly, then a piece of trout. Sprinkle with cilantro and drizzle with lemon juice and oil. Season with salt and pepper. Top fish with orange and lime slices.

2. Bring the long ends of the parchment paper together and fold down until the packet is sealed tightly. Fold up each open end of the paper until the sides of the packet are sealed tightly. Place packets on a baking sheet.

3. Bake in preheated oven for 20 to 30 minutes or until fish is opaque and flakes easily when tested with a fork.

Orecchiette with Baby Peas and Crab

EYE NUTRIENTS: Lutein, zeaxanthin, vitamin C, vitamin E, omega-3s (DHA and EPA), fiber

MAKES 2 SERVINGS

You can use any type of pasta for this dish, but I particularly like it with orecchiette. The combination of vegetables and crab makes it an eye-nutrient powerhouse, and lemon zest and juice give it a pleasant tanginess and a boost of vitamin C.

TIPS: This dish can be served hot, cold or even at room temperature.

You can increase the amount of lemon zest and juice for a zestier version.

VARIATIONS: Substitute ¼ cup (60 mL) sliced green onions for the capers.

This dish tastes great with a bit of spice to liven it up. Add finely chopped hot chile peppers to taste with the onion.

2 tbsp	olive oil	30 mL
½	onion, chopped	½
1	orange or red bell pepper, sliced	1
1 cup	frozen green peas	250 mL
1	can (6 oz/170 g) backfin (lump) crabmeat	1
1 tbsp	chopped fresh parsley or mint (or 1 tsp/5 mL dried)	15 mL
1 tbsp	drained capers	15 mL
	Grated zest and juice of 1 lemon	
	Salt and freshly ground black pepper	
6 oz	dried whole wheat orecchiette pasta (2 cups/500 mL)	175 g
	Lemon-infused olive oil (optional)	

1. In a large saucepan, heat oil over medium-high heat. Add onion and cook, stirring, for 3 to 4 minutes or until translucent. Add orange pepper and peas; cook, stirring, for 3 to 4 minutes or until pepper is softened. Add crab, parsley and capers, stirring well. Remove from heat and stir in lemon zest and juice.

2. Meanwhile, in a pot of boiling water, cook orecchiette for about 10 minutes or until al dente. Drain, reserving ½ cup (125 mL) of the cooking liquid.

3. Add pasta to crab mixture and toss to coat, adding cooking liquid if needed to moisten. Serve drizzled with lemon oil, if desired.

Grilled Scallop and Pineapple Skewers

EYE NUTRIENTS: Vitamin C, vitamin E, zinc, omega-3s (DHA and EPA)

MAKES 4 SERVINGS

Although scallops and pineapple aren't rich enough in eye nutrients to be considered eyefoods on their own, this dish is a source of omega-3 fatty acids, zinc, vitamin E and vitamin C. It's a delicious addition to a backyard barbecue.

VARIATION: You can substitute 12 extra-large shrimp, peeled and deveined, for the scallops. Or use a 1½-inch (4 cm) thick salmon fillet, about 6 inches (15 cm) long and 3 inches (7.5 cm) wide, cut into 12 pieces.

Eyefood Focus

Pineapple is a good source of vitamin C and fiber.

• **4 wood or bamboo skewers, soaked for at least 30 minutes**

Marinade

½ cup	olive oil	125 mL
2 tbsp	unseasoned rice vinegar	30 mL
2 tbsp	freshly squeezed lemon juice	30 mL
1 tbsp	rye whiskey	15 mL
¼ tsp	freshly ground black pepper	1 mL

Skewers

4	slices prosciutto	4
16	2-inch (5 cm) cubes pineapple	16
12	sea scallops, side muscles removed	12

Rub

1 tsp	salt	5 mL
1 tsp	freshly ground black pepper	5 mL
½ tsp	chili powder	2 mL
¼ tsp	garlic powder	1 mL
¼ tsp	paprika	1 mL

1. *Marinade:* In a small bowl, combine oil, vinegar, lemon juice, rye and pepper.

2. *Skewers:* Thread one end of a slice of prosciutto onto each skewer, then alternate pineapple and scallops, threading 4 pineapple cubes and 3 scallops onto each skewer and weaving the prosciutto between the scallops and pineapple, like a ribbon. Place skewers in a shallow glass dish or sealable plastic bag and pour in marinade. Cover or seal and refrigerate for 30 minutes.

3. *Rub:* Meanwhile, in a small bowl, combine salt, pepper, chili powder, garlic powder and paprika.

4. Remove skewers from the refrigerator, discard marinade and rub prepared spices into the scallops. Let stand at room temperature for 15 minutes.

5. Meanwhile, preheat barbecue grill to medium.

6. Grill skewers, turning once, for 8 to 10 minutes or until scallops are firm and opaque.

Shrimp Stir-Fry

EYE NUTRIENTS: Lutein, zeaxanthin, vitamin C, vitamin E, zinc, omega-3s (DHA and EPA)

Precooking the broccoli in this recipe ensures that it stays a vibrant green and does not overcook. Soba noodles, popular in Japanese cuisine, are a great gluten-free alternative to pasta and pair well with stir-fries.

12 oz	dried soba noodles or whole wheat linguine pasta	375 g
	Olive oil	
2 cups	broccoli florets	500 mL
1½ lbs	large shrimp, peeled and deveined	750 g
2	orange bell peppers, sliced	2
1	clove garlic, minced	1
1 tbsp	grated gingerroot	15 mL
4	heads baby bok choy, bottom cut off and leaves separated	4
2	green onions, diagonally sliced	2

Sauce

¼ cup	ready-to-use vegetable broth	60 mL
¼ cup	soy sauce	60 mL
3 tbsp	unseasoned rice vinegar	45 mL
2 tbsp	pure maple syrup	30 mL
1 tbsp	freshly squeezed lime juice	15 mL
1 tbsp	cornstarch	15 mL
¼ cup	cold water	60 mL
	Salt and freshly ground black pepper	

1. In a large pot of boiling salted water, cook soba noodles according to package instructions. Drain, return to the pot, drizzle lightly with oil and stir to coat. Keep warm.

2. *Sauce:* Meanwhile, in a small saucepan, combine broth, soy sauce, vinegar, maple syrup and lime juice. Bring to a boil over medium heat.

3. In a small bowl, combine cornstarch and cold water, stirring to dissolve cornstarch. Add to sauce and season to taste with salt and pepper; return to a boil, stirring constantly. Boil, stirring, for about 2 minutes or until sauce is thickened. Remove from heat and set aside.

4. In a saucepan of boiling water, blanch broccoli florets for 1 minute. Drain and plunge into a bowl of ice water until cool, then drain and set aside.

5. In a wok or large skillet, heat 1 tbsp (15 mL) oil over high heat. Working in batches, add shrimp and stir-fry for 2 to 3 minutes or until pink, firm and opaque. Using a slotted spoon, transfer shrimp to a plate as they are cooked. Repeat with the remaining shrimp, adding more oil and adjusting heat as needed between batches.

6. Add 1 tbsp (15 mL) oil to the wok. Add orange pepper, garlic, ginger and bok choy; stir-fry for 1 minute. Add broccoli and stir-fry for 1 minute. Stir in soba noodles and sauce. Add shrimp and toss gently until heated through. Serve immediately, garnished with green onions.

Chicken Cacciatore

EYE NUTRIENTS: Beta-carotene, lutein, zeaxanthin, vitamin C, vitamin E, zinc

Cacciatore means "hunter" in Italian, and this traditional hunter's stew is typically made with onions and herbs, and often tomatoes and bell peppers. Serve it with whole wheat penne or crusty whole wheat bread or over polenta.

TIP: For mild heat, use about ½ tsp (2 mL) hot pepper flakes, or increase the amount to taste.

Eyefood Focus

Cooked tomatoes are a good source of lycopene, a bright red carotenoid that may have antioxidant effects in the body. Other sources of lycopene include watermelon and papayas.

2 tbsp	all-purpose flour	30 mL
2	boneless skinless chicken breasts (each about 10 oz/300 g), each cut into quarters	2
3 tbsp	olive oil, divided	45 mL
1	orange bell pepper, sliced	1
1	red bell pepper, sliced	1
1	clove garlic, minced	1
½	onion, chopped	½
¾ cup	sliced black olives	175 mL
½ cup	dry red wine	125 mL
2 tbsp	chopped fresh parsley	30 mL
	Hot pepper flakes (see tip)	
1	can (28 oz/796 mL) diced tomatoes, with juice	1
3 tbsp	pumpkin purée (not pie filling)	45 mL
2 tbsp	tomato paste	30 mL
	Salt and freshly ground black pepper	

1. Place flour in a large bowl. Add chicken and turn to coat. Discard any excess flour.

2. In a large saucepan, heat 2 tbsp (30 mL) oil over medium-high heat. Add chicken and sear, turning once, for about 5 minutes or until golden brown on both sides. Transfer chicken to a plate.

3. Add the remaining oil to the pan. Add orange pepper, red pepper, garlic, onion and olives; cook, stirring, for 3 to 5 minutes or until peppers are softened. Stir in wine, scraping up any browned bits from the bottom of the pan.

4. Return chicken and any accumulated juices to the saucepan. Stir in parsley, hot pepper flakes to taste, tomatoes, pumpkin and tomato paste; cover and simmer gently, stirring occasionally, for 18 to 20 minutes or until an instant-read thermometer inserted into the thickest part of a breast registers 165°F (74°C). Season to taste with salt and black pepper.

Chicken and Almond Lettuce Wraps

EYE NUTRIENTS: Lutein, zeaxanthin, vitamin C, vitamin E, zinc

MAKES 4 SERVINGS

This easy dish can be enjoyed as a main course for lunch or served as an appetizer at a dinner party. Have each person assemble their own wraps, for extra fun. This recipe is loaded with both lutein and zeaxanthin.

TIPS: As an appetizer, the wraps serve 8 people. Use 8 lettuce or kale leaves and serve 1 wrap per person.

You can prepare the chicken mixture while the chicken is still hot and enjoy the wraps warm, or you can use cooled or chilled cooked chicken and enjoy them cold.

The chicken mixture and sauce can be prepared through step 3 and refrigerated separately for up to 2 days.

For a zeaxanthin boost, garnish with goji berries.

VARIATIONS: Use 14 oz (400 g) leftover cooked turkey breast in place of the chicken.

Substitute a mango for the orange, and mint for the cilantro.

Replace the dipping sauce with the peanut sauce on page 211.

20 oz	boneless skinless chicken breasts, cooked and pulled into bite-size pieces	600 g
2	green onions, chopped	2
1	large orange, peeled, quartered and sliced	1
1	orange bell pepper, chopped	1
1 cup	frozen peas, thawed	250 mL
1/4 cup	sliced almonds	60 mL
1/4 cup	chopped fresh cilantro	60 mL
8 to 12	leaf or romaine lettuce leaves or kale leaves	8 to 12

Dipping Sauce

1/4 cup	natural almond or peanut butter	60 mL
4 tsp	soy sauce	20 mL
1 tbsp	liquid honey	15 mL
2 tsp	unseasoned rice vinegar	10 mL
Dash	hot pepper sauce	Dash
2 to 3 tbsp	hot water (approx.)	30 to 45 mL

1. In a large serving bowl, combine chicken, green onions, orange, orange pepper, peas, almonds and cilantro.

2. *Sauce:* In a small bowl, combine almond butter, soy sauce, honey, vinegar and hot pepper sauce. Add 2 tbsp (30 mL) hot water and stir well. If sauce is too thick, stir in more hot water until sauce has the consistency of a thick salad dressing.

3. Add 2 tbsp (30 mL) sauce to the chicken mixture and toss gently to combine.

4. Spoon the remaining dipping sauce into individual bowls or ramekins for each person.

5. For each wrap, spoon chicken mixture onto a lettuce leaf and wrap lettuce around chicken mixture. Enjoy with dipping sauce.

Eyefood Focus

Regularly choose whole foods over processed foods and you'll likely consume fewer calories. For example, an orange bell pepper has about 30 calories and is loaded with micronutrients such as vitamin C, zeaxanthin and lutein, whereas a white bagel has about 300 calories and much less nutritional value.

Chicken and Black Bean Rice Bowls with Wasabi Lime Sauce

EYE NUTRIENTS: Lutein, zeaxanthin, vitamin C, vitamin E, zinc, fiber

MAKES 4 SERVINGS

Bowls are appearing on the menus of many restaurants. They are a fun, tasty way to incorporate vegetables, protein and whole grains into a one-dish meal. This version has a spicy kick, thanks to the wasabi in the sauce. Peas, broccoli, spinach and orange peppers make it an eyefoods superstar.

TIPS: If you can only find smaller cans of beans, buy 2 cans, drain and rinse the beans, then measure out 2 cups (500 mL). Store the remaining beans in an airtight container in the refrigerator for up to 3 days.

Do not add salt to this dish, as even reduced-sodium soy sauce is quite salty.

Adjust the wasabi to taste, as it can have quite a bite.

VARIATIONS: Use 14 oz (400 g) leftover cooked turkey breast, chopped, in place of the chicken and add it with the beans.

Substitute cooked barley, quinoa, bulgur or soba noodles for the brown rice.

Wasabi Lime Sauce

1 tbsp	all-purpose flour or cornstarch	15 mL
2 tsp	wasabi powder	10 mL
	Freshly ground black pepper	
	Grated zest of 1 lime	
2 tbsp	freshly squeezed lime juice	30 mL
2 tbsp	liquid honey	30 mL
2 tbsp	reduced-sodium soy sauce	30 mL
2 tbsp	unseasoned rice vinegar or apple cider vinegar	30 mL

Rice Bowls

2 tbsp	olive oil	30 mL
½	onion, chopped	½
1	small clove garlic, minced (or ¼ tsp/1 mL garlic powder)	1
20 oz	boneless skinless chicken breasts, chopped	600 g
1	orange bell pepper, sliced	1
1 cup	broccoli florets	250 mL
1 cup	frozen green peas, thawed	250 mL
1	can (19 oz/540 mL) black beans, drained and rinsed	1
4 cups	packed spinach leaves	1 L
2 cups	hot cooked brown basmati rice (see page 178)	500 mL

1. *Sauce:* In a small bowl, whisk together flour, wasabi powder, pepper to taste, lime zest, lime juice, honey, soy sauce and vinegar (or add ingredients to a jar, seal and shake to combine).

2. *Rice Bowls:* In a large saucepan, heat oil over medium-high heat. Add onion and garlic; cook, stirring, for 2 to 3 minutes or until onion is translucent. Add chicken and cook, stirring, for 8 to 10 minutes or until no longer pink inside. Add orange pepper, broccoli and peas; cook, stirring, for 2 minutes or until broccoli is tender-crisp.

3. Stir in beans. Stir or shake sauce and stir into pan; bring to a simmer, stirring. Simmer, stirring often, for about 5 minutes or until sauce is thickened. Add spinach and stir until wilted (do not overcook).

4. Divide rice among four bowls and spoon chicken mixture over top.

Turkey Stir-Fry with Peanut Sauce

EYE NUTRIENTS: Lutein, vitamin C, vitamin E, zinc

Peanut sauce gives this stir-fry a Thai flair. For the healthiest version, buy natural peanut butter with peanuts as the only ingredient. Serve the stir-fry atop a bed of brown rice or soba noodles.

TIPS: Peanut sauce is common in Thai cuisine. It tastes great as a dip for chicken or a sauce for any stir-fry. Try it as a dipping sauce for Chicken and Almond Lettuce Wraps (page 209).

For a low-carbohydrate meal, serve this stir-fry atop a bed of spinach. The heat from the stir-fry will cause the spinach to cook slightly and wilt.

VARIATION: Replace the rice vinegar in the sauce with freshly squeezed lime juice.

Peanut Sauce

¼ cup	natural peanut butter	60 mL
4 tsp	soy sauce	20 mL
4 tsp	liquid honey	20 mL
2 tsp	unseasoned rice vinegar	10 mL
Dash	hot pepper sauce	Dash
1 to 2 tbsp	hot water	15 to 30 mL

Stir-Fry

2 tbsp	olive oil	30 mL
12 oz	boneless skinless turkey breast, cut into thin strips	375 g
½	red onion, cut into thin wedges	½
1	red bell pepper, sliced	1
2 cups	broccoli florets	500 mL
1 cup	trimmed snow peas	250 mL
2 tbsp	chopped unsalted peanuts	30 mL

1. *Sauce:* In a small bowl, combine peanut butter, soy sauce, honey, vinegar and hot pepper sauce. Add 1 tbsp (15 mL) hot water and stir well. If sauce is too thick, stir in the remaining hot water.

2. *Stir-Fry:* In a wok or large skillet, heat oil over medium-high heat. Working in batches as necessary, add turkey and stir-fry for about 5 minutes or until no longer pink inside. Using a slotted spoon, transfer turkey to a bowl as it is cooked.

3. Add onion to the wok and stir-fry for about 3 minutes or until tender. Add red pepper, broccoli and snow peas; stir-fry for 3 to 5 minutes or until vegetables are tender-crisp and vibrant in color.

4. Return turkey and any accumulated juices to the wok, stirring well. Remove from heat and stir in peanut sauce. Serve garnished with peanuts.

Turkey Fajitas

EYE NUTRIENTS: Lutein, zeaxanthin, vitamin C, vitamin E, zinc

	MAKES 4 SERVINGS	

Fajitas are a regular meal in my house. They are fun to eat and nutritious. Turkey breast gives a boost of zinc and vitamin E, and green onions contribute lutein. You can include bell peppers in any colors, but remember that orange peppers have the most zeaxanthin and lutein.

TIPS: To warm the tortillas, microwave each one on Medium for 5 seconds.

Assembled fajitas also taste great grilled in a panini press.

VARIATION: Substitute lean beef strips for the turkey breast.

1 tbsp	olive oil	15 mL
1½ lbs	boneless skinless turkey breast or chicken breasts, cut into long strips	750 g
¼ cup	ready-to-use chicken broth or water (optional)	60 mL
¼	Spanish or Vidalia onion, cut into long strips	¼
3 tbsp	chili powder	45 mL
1 tsp	ground cumin	5 mL
2 tbsp	freshly squeezed lime juice	30 mL
1	orange bell pepper, sliced lengthwise	1
½	red bell pepper, sliced lengthwise	½
1 cup	frozen corn kernels	250 mL
½ cup	rinsed drained canned black beans	125 mL
4	green onions, cut into long strips	4
	Salt and freshly ground black pepper	
	Cayenne pepper or hot pepper sauce (optional)	
8	12-inch (30 cm) whole-grain flour or corn tortillas, warmed	8

Garnishes

Chopped fresh cilantro

Sour cream

Shredded Cheddar cheese

Salsa

Minced jalapeño peppers

1. In a large skillet, heat oil over high heat. Add turkey and cook, stirring, for 2 minutes. If turkey starts to stick, add broth and scrape up browned bits from the bottom of the pan. Add onion and cook, stirring, for 5 to 7 minutes or until turkey is no longer pink inside and onion is tender. Add chili powder, cumin and lime juice, stirring well.

2. Stir in orange pepper, red pepper, corn and beans; cook, stirring, for 3 to 5 minutes or until peppers have softened. Season to taste with salt, black pepper and cayenne (if using). Transfer to a serving bowl.

3. Place each garnish in its own bowl and stack warmed tortillas on a plate. Arrange all of the fajita fixings on the table and let diners assemble their own fajitas.

Turkey, Pea and Carrot Barley Bowls

EYE NUTRIENTS: Beta-carotene, lutein, vitamin C, vitamin E, zinc, fiber

MAKES 2 SERVINGS

Here's a modern twist on the classic peas and carrots dish. It's a good way to use up leftover turkey or chicken after a big festive dinner (see tip).

TIPS: If using leftovers to create this dish, just heat the oil and sauté any uncooked ingredients, then add the leftovers and sauté until reheated.

Other leftovers you could incorporate include sweet potato or butternut squash in place of the carrots, and Brussels sprouts or cauliflower in place of the peas.

VARIATION: Substitute any cooked whole grain for the barley. Good options are quinoa, brown rice or buckwheat.

1 tbsp	olive oil	15 mL
12 oz	boneless skinless turkey breast or chicken breasts, cut into strips	375 g
3	carrots, chopped	3
1 cup	frozen green peas, thawed	250 mL
1 tbsp	grated gingerroot (or 2 tsp/10 mL ground ginger)	15 mL
	Salt and freshly ground black pepper	
1 cup	hot cooked barley (see page 178)	250 mL

1. In a large saucepan, heat oil over medium-high heat. Add turkey and cook, stirring, for 8 to 10 minutes or until no longer pink inside. Add carrots, peas and ginger; cook, stirring, for 5 minutes or until carrots are tender. Season to taste with salt and pepper.

2. Divide barley between two bowls and spoon turkey mixture over top.

Eyefoods Shepherd's Pie

EYE NUTRIENTS: Beta-carotene, lutein, zeaxanthin, vitamin C, vitamin E, zinc, fiber

MAKES 4 TO 6 SERVINGS

This eye-friendly version of shepherd's pie uses turkey in place of beef or lamb, and sweet potatoes instead of white potatoes. It contains a high amount of beta-carotene and zinc, and the spinach and peas add lutein.

VARIATION: Substitute cooked chopped kale for the spinach. You'll need about 3½ oz (100 g) chopped trimmed kale to get 1 cup (250 mL) cooked.

Eyefood Focus

Turkey is a great source of zinc and vitamin E. As a low-fat source of protein, it's an important part of an eye-healthy diet.

- **Preheat oven to 375°F (190°C)**
- **9-inch (23 cm) square baking pan**

2	sweet potatoes (about 12 oz/375 g total), peeled and cut into quarters	2
	Water	
2 tbsp	olive oil	30 mL
1	small onion, chopped	1
1	clove garlic, minced	1
1 lb	extra-lean ground turkey	500 g
1 cup	frozen chopped spinach (3½ oz/100 g or 6 cubes)	250 mL
2 cups	frozen green peas, thawed	500 mL
1 tbsp	chopped fresh parsley (or 1 tsp/5 mL dried)	15 mL
1 tbsp	chopped fresh sage (or 1 tsp/5 mL dried)	15 mL
¼ tsp	cayenne pepper (optional)	1 mL
	Salt and freshly ground black pepper	
¼ cup	dry white wine	60 mL
1 tbsp	Dijon mustard	15 mL
¼ cup	milk	60 mL
2 tbsp	pure maple syrup	30 mL
¼ tsp	ground cinnamon	1 mL
¼ cup	shredded Cheddar cheese (optional)	60 mL

1. Place sweet potatoes in a medium saucepan and add enough water to cover. Cover and bring to a boil over high heat. Uncover and boil for 20 to 30 minutes or until fork-tender.

2. Meanwhile, in a large saucepan, heat oil over medium-high heat. Add onion and garlic; cook, stirring, for 1 to 2 minutes or until onion is softened. Add turkey and cook, stirring and breaking it up with a spoon, for about 8 minutes or until no longer pink. Add frozen spinach and cook until it breaks up and integrates into the turkey mixture. Add peas, parsley, sage, cayenne (if using), salt and black pepper to taste, wine and mustard; reduce heat and simmer, stirring occasionally, for 10 minutes. Transfer to baking pan.

3. Drain sweet potatoes, return to the pan and add milk, maple syrup, cinnamon, and salt and pepper to taste; use a potato masher to mash sweet potatoes to a smooth consistency. Spread over turkey mixture. Cover with foil.

4. Bake in preheated oven for 25 minutes. Uncover, sprinkle with cheese (if using) and bake for 5 minutes or until cheese is melted.

Turkey Burgers with Roasted Orange Peppers

EYE NUTRIENTS: Lutein, zeaxanthin, vitamin C, vitamin E, zinc, fiber

MAKES 4 SERVINGS

These yummy turkey burgers will turn your weekend barbecue into an eye-healthy feast. Turkey is high in zinc, and orange peppers and green onion provide lutein and zeaxanthin.

TIPS: When you let grilled (or roasted) peppers cool inside a paper bag, the steam helps separate the skin from the flesh, making the peppers easier to peel.

Caramelize onions by cooking thinly sliced onions in olive oil in a skillet over low heat, stirring often, for about 20 minutes or until very tender. Season with salt and pepper. Serve as a topping for the burgers.

VARIATION: For a lighter version, omit the buns and serve the turkey patties wrapped in lettuce leaves.

- Preheat barbecue grill to high
- 4 squares parchment paper

1 lb	extra-lean ground turkey	500 g
1	large omega-3 egg, beaten	1
½ cup	chopped green onions	125 mL
¼ cup	dry whole wheat bread crumbs or oat bran	60 mL
¼ cup	chopped fresh flat-leaf (Italian) parsley	60 mL
	Salt and freshly ground black pepper	
2	orange bell peppers	2
3 tbsp	grainy Dijon mustard	45 mL
4	whole wheat burger buns, split	4
	Leaf lettuce	

1. In a large bowl, combine turkey, egg, green onions, bread crumbs and parsley. Season with salt and pepper. Form into four ½-inch (1 cm) thick patties. Place each patty on a square of parchment paper and refrigerate while you prepare the peppers.

2. Place peppers on preheated grill and grill, turning, for 15 to 20 minutes or until charred on all sides. Remove from grill, place in a paper bag, close tightly and let cool for 10 minutes. Decrease grill heat to medium.

3. Working over a bowl to collect the juices, peel peppers and discard skins. Cut peppers into wedges and discard stems, seeds and membranes.

4. Mix 1 tbsp (15 mL) pepper juice with mustard.

5. Holding on to the parchment paper, flip turkey patties over onto the grill, remove the paper and cook, turning once, for 5 to 6 minutes per side or until an instant-read thermometer inserted horizontally into a patty registers at least 165°F (74°C).

6. When patties are almost ready, toast burger buns on the grill.

7. Spread mustard mixture on cut sides of buns. Divide roasted pepper wedges evenly among bottom halves of buns, top each with a turkey patty and lettuce, then cover with top halves of buns.

Turkey Meatballs in Tomato Sauce

EYE NUTRIENTS: Vitamin E, zinc, fiber

MAKES 4 SERVINGS

I may be a bit biased, but I truly believe my mom makes the most delicious meatballs. When I asked her to create an eye-healthy version, she came up with a recipe that rivals the original. It uses turkey in place of beef and pork, and includes wheat germ for an added dose of fiber and vitamin E. After slow-simmering in tomato sauce, these meatballs are fantastic over cooked whole wheat pasta or packed into a whole wheat sub roll, for a satisfying comfort-food meal.

TIPS: For small cocktail-size meatballs, form the meat mixture into 20 small meatballs. After step 1, arrange meatballs on a rimmed baking sheet lined with parchment paper and bake in a 400°F (200°C) oven for 20 to 25 minutes or until no longer pink inside.

The cooked meatballs freeze well. You can make larger batches and freeze them, either in pasta sauce or on their own, for up to 3 months.

1 lb	extra-lean ground turkey	500 g
2	large omega-3 eggs, beaten	2
1	clove garlic, minced	1
¼ cup	wheat germ	60 mL
¼ cup	dry whole wheat bread crumbs	60 mL
¼ cup	freshly grated Parmesan cheese	60 mL
2 tbsp	chopped fresh parsley (or 1 tbsp/15 mL dried)	30 mL
	Salt and freshly ground black pepper	
1 tbsp	olive oil	15 mL
3 cups	tomato pasta sauce	750 mL

1. In a large bowl, combine turkey, eggs, garlic, wheat germ, bread crumbs, cheese and parsley. Season with salt and pepper. Form into 12 large meatballs.

2. In a large saucepan, heat oil over high heat. Add meatballs and sear, turning often, for 2 to 3 minutes or until browned on all sides.

3. Add tomato sauce, reduce heat and simmer for 15 to 20 minutes or until meatballs are no longer pink inside.

Stuffed Orange Peppers

EYE NUTRIENTS: Beta-carotene, lutein, zeaxanthin, vitamin C, vitamin E, zinc, fiber

My eye-healthy version of stuffed peppers uses barley in place of rice. Orange peppers make this dish an excellent source of zeaxanthin and vitamin C, and the spinach and eggs contribute extra lutein.

TIPS: This recipe will produce peppers with a firm texture. If you prefer more tender peppers, precook them in a 350°F (180°C) oven for 10 minutes before stuffing.

Make extra turkey mixture and freeze it in an airtight container for up to 3 months. Thaw overnight, then stuff the peppers and bake, for a quick, tasty supper.

VARIATIONS: For a vegetarian version, replace the meat with 1 cup (250 mL) cooked or canned black beans or chickpeas.

Use 1 cup (250 mL) chopped trimmed raw kale in place of the spinach to increase the amount of lutein.

Add ¼ cup (60 mL) pine nuts or chopped dried apricots to the stuffing.

- Preheat oven to 375°F (190°C)
- 6-cup (1.5 L) casserole dish

1 tbsp	olive oil	15 mL
8 oz	extra-lean ground turkey or beef	250 g
1 or 2	cloves garlic, minced	1 or 2
1	carrot, chopped	1
1	stalk celery, chopped	1
¼	onion, chopped	¼
¼ cup	frozen chopped spinach (1½ cubes)	60 mL
1 tsp	dried Italian seasoning	5 mL
1 tsp	dried sage	5 mL
1 cup	cooked barley (see page 178)	250 mL
1	large omega-3 egg, beaten	1
4	orange bell peppers	4
2 cups	tomato sauce	500 mL
¾ cup	ready-to-use chicken broth	175 mL
	Salt and freshly ground black pepper	

1. In a large saucepan, heat oil over medium-high heat. Add turkey and cook, breaking it up with a spoon, for 3 to 5 minutes or until no longer pink.

2. Add garlic to taste, carrot, celery and onion; cook, stirring, for 5 minutes or until tender. Add frozen spinach, Italian seasoning and sage; cook, stirring, until spinach has softened. Drain off excess fat. Stir in barley. Remove from heat and let cool, then add egg and stir to combine well.

3. Remove tops and seeds from orange peppers. Fill peppers with turkey mixture, dividing evenly.

4. In casserole dish, combine tomato sauce and broth, stirring well. Stand peppers upright in dish. Cover with foil.

5. Bake in preheated oven for about 1 hour or until peppers are fork-tender.

Mom's Eye-Friendly Meatloaf

EYE NUTRIENTS: Beta-carotene, lutein, zeaxanthin, vitamin E, zinc

When I asked my mom to create a meatloaf that included eyefoods, she came up with this delicious recipe. It's a great source of vitamin E and zinc, and she even managed to sneak in some lutein with the addition of spinach.

TIPS: To save time, double this recipe and make two meatloaves at once. You can serve the second as leftovers later in the week. Mix it up by making meatloaf sandwiches with thin slices of meatloaf, whole-grain bread, Dijon mustard and romaine lettuce.

Leftover sliced meatloaf can be stored in an airtight container in the refrigerator for up to 3 days.

- Preheat oven to 350°F (180°C)
- 9- by 5-inch (23 by 12.5 cm) loaf pan, lined with lightly greased parchment paper

1 lb	lean ground beef	500 g
1 lb	extra-lean ground turkey	500 g
2	large omega-3 eggs, beaten	2
1	package (10 oz/284 g) chopped frozen spinach, thawed and excess liquid squeezed out	1
½	onion, chopped	½
½ cup	chopped carrots	125 mL
½ cup	freshly grated Parmesan cheese	125 mL
½ cup	dry whole wheat bread crumbs	125 mL

1. In a large bowl, combine beef, turkey, eggs, spinach, onion, carrots, cheese and bread crumbs. Pack into prepared pan.

2. Bake in preheated oven for 1½ hours or until an instant-read thermometer inserted in the center registers at least 165°F (74°C).

Beef and Broccoli with Barley

EYE NUTRIENTS: Lutein, zeaxanthin, vitamin C, vitamin E, zinc, fiber

If you prepare barley ahead of time, this delicious weeknight meal comes together quickly. I like to make it a bit spicy, but you can adjust the amount of wasabi to your taste. I often mix soy sauce and wasabi in a separate bowl so everyone can add it to their plate according to their palate; if you do this, omit the wasabi from step 1.

TIP: Allocate a few hours once a week to meal prep. Blanch vegetables, such as broccoli and green beans; cook whole grains, such as barley, brown rice or quinoa; and sauté lean beef or turkey breast strips. Having these healthy options prepared and ready to go in the fridge makes weeknight meal assembly quick and easy.

2 tbsp	soy sauce	30 mL
2 tbsp	ready-to-use reduced-sodium beef broth	30 mL
2 tbsp	freshly squeezed lime juice	30 mL
1/4 tsp	wasabi powder	1 mL
2 tbsp	olive oil	30 mL
8 oz	lean beef (such as tenderloin or sirloin), cut into strips	250 g
4 cups	broccoli florets and chopped peeled stems	1 L
1 tbsp	grated gingerroot	15 mL
1 tbsp	chopped fresh cilantro	15 mL
2 cups	hot cooked barley (see page 178)	500 mL

1. In a medium bowl, combine soy sauce, broth, lime juice and wasabi. Set aside.

2. In a large skillet, heat oil over high heat. Add beef and cook, stirring, for 1 to 2 minutes or until browned on all sides but still pink inside. Add broccoli, ginger, cilantro and soy sauce mixture; reduce heat to medium-high and cook, stirring, for 3 to 5 minutes or until broccoli is tender but still vibrant in color. Add barley and cook for 1 minute, stirring well.

Mango and Beef Stir-Fry

EYE NUTRIENTS: Lutein, zeaxanthin, vitamin C, vitamin E, zinc

MAKES 4 SERVINGS

Stir-fries are an excellent way to include a lot of vegetables in your diet, so pull out your wok! Once you start, you'll be inspired to stir-fry more often and to try different combinations of veggies and protein. If you don't have a wok, you can use a large skillet. The key to a great stir-fry is to cook over high heat and make sure the pan isn't crowded.

TIPS: Thai basil has slender pointed oval leaves and a distinct anise flavor. It is popular in Asian cuisines. If you cannot find Thai basil, you can substitute cilantro. Cilantro has a very different flavor than Thai basil, but it also works well in this dish.

This stir-fry tastes great atop brown basmati rice or quinoa.

Sauce

1 to 2 tbsp	minced gingerroot	15 to 30 mL
2 tbsp	reduced-sodium soy sauce	30 mL
2 tbsp	orange juice	30 mL
1 tbsp	unseasoned rice vinegar	15 mL
1 tbsp	freshly squeezed lemon juice	15 mL
1 tbsp	pure maple syrup	15 mL
1 tsp	hot pepper sauce	5 mL

Stir-Fry

1 tbsp	olive oil	15 mL
1 lb	lean beef (such as sirloin or strip loin), cut into strips	500 g
4	green onions, sliced	4
2	orange bell peppers, sliced lengthwise	2
2	mangos, sliced lengthwise	2
¼ cup	chopped fresh parsley	60 mL
¼ cup	chopped fresh Thai basil (see tip)	60 mL

1. *Sauce:* In a small bowl, whisk together ginger to taste, soy sauce, orange juice, vinegar, lemon juice, maple syrup and hot pepper sauce. Set aside.

2. *Stir-Fry:* In a wok or large skillet, heat oil over medium-high heat. Working in batches as necessary, add beef and stir-fry for 5 to 8 minutes or until cooked as desired. Using a slotted spoon, transfer beef to a bowl as it is cooked.

3. Add green onions and orange peppers to the wok and stir-fry for 3 to 5 minutes or until peppers are tender-crisp but still vibrant in color.

4. Return beef and any accumulated juices to the wok, stirring well. Stir in sauce and cook for 2 minutes. Remove from heat and stir in mangos, parsley and Thai basil.

Healthy Snacks and Desserts

It's not always easy to make healthy snack choices, but you can make it easier by having eye-friendly snacks prepared and ready in your pantry or fridge. In addition to some nut, seed and dried fruit mixes, I have provided three recipes for kale chips, a very popular snack option and a good way to introduce children to kale. I'm always surprised by how many children love kale chips.

As you start to follow the Eyefoods Plan, you will find yourself eating a lot more vegetables, including broccoli, orange peppers, carrots and zucchini. This chapter also includes recipes for healthy dips to liven up your raw veggies.

The dessert recipes are low in sugar and have the added benefits of eye-healthy nutrients. The pumpkin mousse is a good source of beta-carotene, while the sabayon is an excellent source of lutein.

Snacks

Eyefoods Nut Mix 222
Eyefoods Trail Mix 222
Eyefoods Granola. 223
Kale Chips 223
Nutty Kale Chips 224
Seedy Kale Chips 225
Pickled Peppers 225
Mini Pepper Sailboats 226
Hummus 226
Pumpkin Hummus 227
White Bean Dip 227

Desserts

Pumpkin Mousse 228
Sabayon with Fresh Fruit 229

Eyefoods Nut Mix

EYE NUTRIENTS: Vitamin E, zinc, omega-3s (ALA)

MAKES 3½ CUPS (875 ML)

This quick and easy snack contains a balance of the eye nutrients found in nuts. Make a large jar of this nut mix and enjoy a handful each day. It is also a great snack for a party, and the foundation of Eyefoods Trail Mix (below) and Eyefoods Granola (page 223).

TIP: Choose unsalted nuts for the healthiest version of this mix.

1 cup	green pumpkin seeds (pepitas)	250 mL
1 cup	chopped almonds	250 mL
1 cup	chopped cashews	250 mL
½ cup	chopped walnuts	125 mL

1. In a large glass jar or storage container, combine pumpkin seeds, almonds, cashews and walnuts. Store in a cool, dry place for up to 2 weeks.

> **Eyefood Focus**
> Nuts are a healthy snack choice, but they are calorie-dense and can lead to weight gain if you eat too many. Consume 1 handful of nuts per day.

Eyefoods Trail Mix

EYE NUTRIENTS: Beta-carotene, zeaxanthin, vitamin E, zinc, omega-3s (ALA)

MAKES 3½ CUPS (875 ML)

Add some pizzazz to your nut mix and satisfy your sweet tooth by adding some dried fruit. This is a great snack to pack for a hike or a long car ride.

2 cups	Eyefoods Nut Mix (above)	500 mL
1 cup	dried apricots, chopped	250 mL
½ cup	dried goji berries	125 mL

1. In a large glass jar or storage container, combine nut mix, apricots and goji berries. Store in a cool, dry place for up to 2 weeks.

Eyefoods Granola

EYE NUTRIENTS: Beta-carotene, zeaxanthin, vitamin E, zinc, omega-3s (ALA), fiber

MAKES 8 CUPS (2 L)

Enjoy this granola as a snack, for breakfast or even for dessert. Like the Eyefoods Trail Mix (page 222), it is easy to store and great to pack along when hiking, camping or backpacking.

TIP: For breakfast, enjoy this granola with milk. Or sprinkle it over yogurt and add fresh fruit to make a tasty parfait that you can enjoy for breakfast or dessert.

- Preheat oven to 350°F (180°C)
- Candy/deep-fry thermometer

4 cups	large-flake (old-fashioned) rolled oats	1 L
1 cup	pure maple syrup	250 mL
2 tbsp	butter	30 mL
1 cup	wheat germ	250 mL
2 cups	Eyefoods Trail Mix (page 222)	500 mL

1. Spread oats on a baking sheet and toast in preheated oven for 10 minutes. Stir and continue toasting for 5 minutes.

2. Meanwhile, in a small saucepan, bring maple syrup and butter to a boil over high heat. Boil for about 10 minutes or until a candy thermometer registers 234°F (112°C).

3. In large bowl, combine toasted oats, wheat germ and trail mix. Add hot maple syrup mixture and stir well.

4. Line the baking sheet with parchment paper. Spread granola out over baking sheet and let cool to room temperature, then break into bite-size pieces.

5. Store in an airtight container in a cool, dry place for up to 2 weeks.

Kale Chips

EYE NUTRIENTS: Beta-carotene, lutein, zeaxanthin, vitamin C, vitamin E, zinc

MAKES 2 TO 4 SERVINGS

This healthy alternative to potato chips is beloved by the choosiest of kids and adults alike!

TIP: The key to this recipe is to bake the kale chips low and slow, to keep them from burning.

- Preheat oven to 250°F (125°C)
- Large rimmed baking sheet, lined with parchment paper

6 cups	trimmed kale leaves (about 5 oz/150 g)	1.5 L
1 tbsp	extra virgin olive oil	15 mL
	Salt and freshly ground black pepper	

1. Remove ribs from kale leaves and roughly chop kale into bite-size pieces.

2. Place kale in a large bowl, drizzle with oil and season to taste with salt and pepper. Using your hands, lightly massage kale to coat evenly. Spread kale in a single layer on prepared baking sheet.

3. Bake in preheated oven for 35 to 45 minutes or until crisp. Enjoy immediately or store in an airtight container for up to 1 week.

Nutty Kale Chips

EYE NUTRIENTS: Beta-carotene, lutein, zeaxanthin, vitamin C, vitamin E, zinc

MAKES 2 TO 4 SERVINGS

Inspired by the "raw" kale chips found in health food stores, these chips have a nutty flavor and a crunchy texture. The cayenne pepper is optional, but if you like spicy foods, it adds real zing.

TIP: Nutritional yeast is a deactivated yeast that comes in the form of flakes or powder. It can be found at health food stores and is popular in vegan and vegetarian diets as a substitute for cheese. It has a nutty, cheesy flavor and can be used as a topping for popcorn or in mashed potatoes.

- Preheat oven to 250°F (120°C)
- Coffee or spice grinder
- Large rimmed baking sheet, lined with parchment paper

Seasoning Blend

2 tbsp	pistachios	30 mL
2 tbsp	sliced almonds	30 mL
⅓ cup	nutritional yeast	75 mL
2 tbsp	wheat germ	30 mL
1 tbsp	paprika	15 mL
Pinch	cayenne pepper (optional)	Pinch
	Finely grated zest of 1 lime	

Kale Chips

6 cups	trimmed kale leaves (about 5 oz/150 g)	1.5 L
¼ tsp	freshly cracked black pepper	1 mL
⅛ tsp	salt	0.5 mL
2 tsp	freshly squeezed lime juice	10 mL

1. *Seasoning Blend:* Using the coffee grinder, grind pistachios and almonds to a fine powder.

2. In a small bowl, combine powdered nuts, yeast, wheat germ, paprika, cayenne (if using) and lime zest. Set aside.

3. *Kale Chips:* Remove ribs from kale leaves and roughly chop kale into bite-size pieces.

4. Place kale in a large bowl and sprinkle with salt, pepper and lime juice. Using your hands, lightly massage kale to coat evenly. Add ¼ cup (60 mL) seasoning blend and toss to coat. Spread kale in a single layer on prepared baking sheet and sprinkle with the remaining seasoning blend.

5. Bake in preheated oven for 35 to 45 minutes or until crisp. Enjoy immediately or store in an airtight container for up to 1 week.

Seedy Kale Chips

EYE NUTRIENTS: Beta-carotene, lutein, zeaxanthin, vitamin C, vitamin E, zinc

MAKES 2 TO 4 SERVINGS

Sunflower seeds, pumpkin seeds and wheat germ give these kale chips crunch and increase their vitamin E and zinc content.

Eyefood Focus

Kale is not only good for your eyes, it is often celebrated for its protective properties against cardiovascular disease and cancer.

- Preheat oven to 250°F (120°C)
- Small food processor or mini chopper
- Large rimmed baking sheet, lined with parchment paper

6 cups	trimmed kale leaves (about 5 oz/150 g)	1.5 L
2 tbsp	sunflower seeds	30 mL
2 tbsp	green pumpkin seeds (pepitas)	30 mL
2 tbsp	wheat germ	30 mL
2 tbsp	nutritional yeast	30 mL
1 tbsp	olive oil	15 mL

1. Remove ribs from kale leaves and roughly chop kale into bite-size pieces.

2. In food processor, combine sunflower seeds, pumpkin seeds, wheat germ and yeast; process to a grainy consistency.

3. Place kale in a large bowl, drizzle with oil and sprinkle with seed mixture. Using your hands, lightly massage kale to coat evenly. Spread kale in a single layer on prepared baking sheet.

4. Bake in preheated oven for 35 to 45 minutes or until crisp. Enjoy immediately or store in an airtight container for up to 1 week.

Pickled Peppers

EYE NUTRIENTS: Lutein, zeaxanthin, vitamin C, vitamin E

MAKES 2 TO 4 SERVINGS

These peppers are a nice alternative to pickles and are loaded with vitamin C. Enjoy them as a snack, a sandwich topping or a condiment, or toss with olive oil for a nice salad.

2	orange bell peppers, sliced	2
1	red bell pepper, sliced	1
1	yellow bell pepper, sliced	1
1 tbsp	salt	15 mL
1½ cups	apple cider vinegar	375 mL
1½ cups	water	375 mL

1. In a glass or stainless steel bowl, combine orange, red and yellow peppers, salt, vinegar and water, ensuring peppers are covered with liquid. Cover and soak overnight or for up to 3 days.

2. Transfer to an airtight container and store in the refrigerator for up to 1 week.

Mini Pepper Sailboats

EYE NUTRIENTS: Lutein, zeaxanthin, vitamin C, vitamin E, zinc, fiber

MAKES 20 MINI SAILBOATS

These sailboats make it fun for kids to eat orange peppers. They are a great snack for a kids' birthday party.

TIPS: If you cannot find mini orange peppers, cut 5 regular orange bell peppers lengthwise into quarters.

For a simple school lunch, prepare hummus early in the week and assemble the peppers the night before. You may need to omit the sails, or lay them down, to pack the boats up easily.

- **20 toothpicks**

½	zucchini	½
1 cup	Hummus (below)	250 mL
10	mini orange peppers, cut in half, seeds and ribs removed	10

1. Peel zucchini and cut crosswise into 2-inch (5 cm) long pieces, then cut each piece into thin slices, making 20 slices total.

2. Spoon 1 to 2 tsp (5 to 10 mL) hummus into each pepper half. Thread a zucchini slice vertically onto each toothpick, piercing it twice, to create a "sail." Insert a toothpick into each pepper. Arrange sailboats on a platter.

> **Eyefood Focus**
>
> Eating foods high in lutein and zeaxanthin, like orange peppers, can increase your macular pigment, giving you a lower risk of developing a chronic eye disease such as age-related macular degeneration.

Hummus

EYE NUTRIENTS: Vitamin E, zinc, fiber

MAKES ABOUT 1½ CUPS (375 ML)

Chickpeas are the star of this versatile hummus. It is high in protein and fiber and is a great addition to sliced orange peppers, raw broccoli and carrots for a midafternoon snack.

TIP: For a delicious sandwich, spread hummus over whole-grain bread and top with pea sprouts and a mixture of roasted veggies.

- **Food processor**

1	clove garlic, coarsely chopped	1
1 cup	rinsed drained canned chickpeas	250 mL
2 tsp	chili powder	10 mL
1 tbsp	freshly squeezed lime juice	15 mL
¼ cup	extra virgin olive oil	60 mL
	Salt and freshly ground black pepper	

1. In food processor, combine garlic, chickpeas, chili powder and lime juice. While pulsing, gradually add oil through the feed tube and pulse until evenly combined and smooth.

2. Transfer hummus to a bowl and season to taste with salt and pepper. Serve immediately or cover and refrigerate for up to 3 days.

Pumpkin Hummus

EYE NUTRIENTS: Beta-carotene, vitamin E, zinc, fiber

MAKES ABOUT 1¾ CUPS (425 ML)

This hummus packs a punch of beta-carotene thanks to the pumpkin purée. In addition to being a great year-round snack, it makes a great dip to serve with an assortment of raw veggies as an appetizer for Thanksgiving dinner.

- **Food processor**

1	clove garlic, coarsely chopped	1
1 cup	rinsed drained canned chickpeas	250 mL
¼ cup	pumpkin purée (not pie filling)	60 mL
Pinch	hot pepper flakes	Pinch
1 tbsp	freshly squeezed lime juice	15 mL
¼ cup	extra virgin olive oil	60 mL
	Salt and freshly ground black pepper	
	Hot pepper sauce	

1. In food processer, combine garlic, chickpeas, pumpkin, hot pepper flakes and lime juice. While pulsing, gradually add oil through the feed tube and pulse until evenly combined and smooth.

2. Transfer hummus to a bowl and season to taste with salt, black pepper and hot pepper sauce. Serve immediately or cover and refrigerate for up to 3 days.

White Bean Dip

EYE NUTRIENTS: Vitamin E, zinc, fiber

MAKES ABOUT 2½ CUPS (625 ML)

This dip is a staple at my house when I entertain. It is quick to make and high in fiber and zinc. I always make a double batch and keep some in the fridge to enjoy with veggies or as a sandwich spread later in the week.

- **Food processor**

8	drained oil-packed sun-dried tomatoes, coarsely chopped	8
1	clove garlic, coarsely chopped	1
2 cups	rinsed drained canned cannellini (white kidney) beans	500 mL
2 tbsp	freshly squeezed lemon juice	30 mL
2 tbsp	extra virgin olive oil	30 mL
	Salt and freshly ground black pepper	

1. In food processor, combine sun-dried tomatoes, garlic, beans, lemon juice and oil; process until smooth.

2. Transfer to a bowl and season to taste with salt and pepper. Serve immediately or cover and refrigerate for up to 3 days.

Pumpkin Mousse

EYE NUTRIENTS: Beta-carotene, vitamin E

Trade your traditional pumpkin pie for this lighter dessert. Packed with beta-carotene, it will nourish your eyes and satisfy your sweet tooth.

- **Handheld electric mixer**

1 cup	pumpkin purée (not pie filling)	250 mL
½ cup	plain Greek yogurt	125 mL
1	envelope (¼ oz/7 g) unflavored gelatin powder	1
	Grated zest of 1 orange	
¼ cup	freshly squeezed orange juice	60 mL
½ cup	pure maple syrup	125 mL
¼ cup	cold heavy or whipping (35%) cream	60 mL
½ tsp	pumpkin pie spice	2 mL

1. Put a medium bowl in the freezer.

2. In a large bowl, whisk together pumpkin and yogurt.

3. Sprinkle gelatin over orange juice and let stand while you heat the maple syrup.

4. In a small saucepan, bring maple syrup to a boil over medium-high heat, stirring constantly. Pour over orange juice mixture and stir until gelatin has melted.

5. Add maple syrup mixture to pumpkin mixture and whisk until well combined. Stir in orange zest and pumpkin pie spice.

6. In the chilled bowl, using the handheld mixer, whip cream to firm peaks.

7. Using the handheld mixer (no need to clean the beaters), whip pumpkin mixture for 1 minute. Gently fold in whipped cream.

8. Ladle mousse into serving cups and refrigerate for at least 2 hours, until set, or for up to 1 day.

Sabayon with Fresh Fruit

EYE NUTRIENTS: Lutein, vitamin C, vitamin E, zinc, omega-3s (DHA)

MAKES 4 SERVINGS

Sabayon is the French version of the traditional Italian dessert zabaglione. One of my favorite memories is of this dessert being made tableside for me and my husband at a restaurant where we were celebrating our 10th wedding anniversary. I use ice wine for a local twist, as it hails from Ontario's Niagara region, my home, but sweet white wine, champagne, port or sherry can be substituted. Serve with fruits of the season: berries, citrus fruits and kiwifruit are all great eyefoods choices.

TIP: This is a great dessert when you are hosting a dinner party. As everyone gathers in the kitchen, you can prepare it in front of your guests, just before serving.

4	large omega-3 egg yolks	4
3 tbsp	ice wine	45 mL
2 tbsp	pure maple syrup	30 mL
1 cup	fresh fruit (chopped or sliced as necessary)	250 mL

1. Add 1 inch (2.5 cm) water to a medium saucepan and bring to a gentle boil.

2. In a large heatproof bowl, whisk together egg yolks, ice wine and maple syrup. Place bowl over the gently boiling water, making sure the water does not touch the bowl. Cook, whisking constantly to make sure it does not turn into scrambled eggs, for 4 to 6 minutes or until the mixture is tripled in volume and creates a ribbon effect when the whisk is raised. Be careful not to overcook, as the mixture can curdle quite quickly.

3. Transfer sabayon to a small glass bowl and serve warm, or let cool and serve within 4 hours, topped with fruit.

Resources and References

Resources

All About Vision
www.allaboutvision.com

American Academy of Ophthalmology
www.aao.org

American Heart Association
www.heart.org/en/healthy-living/healthy-eating

American Optometric Association
www.aoa.org

Canadian Ophthalmological Society
www.cos-sco.ca

Canadian Association of Optometrists
https://opto.ca

References

References Used Throughout

American Heart Association. Fish and omega-3 fatty acids. Available at: www.heart.org/en/healthy-living/healthy-eating/eat-smart/fats/fish-and-omega-3-fatty-acids. Accessed June 1, 2018.

American Heart Association. How do I follow a healthy diet? *Answers by Heart*, 2015. Available at: www.heart.org/-/media/data-import/downloadables/pe-abh-how-do-i-follow-a-healthy-diet-ucm_300467.pdf. Accessed June 1, 2018.

American Heart Association. Whole grains, refined grains, and dietary fiber. Available at: www.heart.org/en/healthy-living/healthy-eating/eat-smart/nutrition-basics/whole-grains-refined-grains-and-dietary-fiber. Accessed June 1, 2018.

Béliveau R, Gingras D. *Cooking with Foods that Fight Cancer*. Toronto: McClelland & Stewart, 2007.

Canadian Society for Exercise Physiology. Canadian physical activity guidelines. Available at: www.csep.ca/CMFiles/Guidelines/CSEP_PAGuidelines_adults_en.pdf. Accessed June 1, 2018.

Capogna L, Pelletier B. *Eyefoods: A Food Plan for Healthy Eyes*. St. David's, ON: LB Media Concepts Inc., 2011.

Canadian Cancer Society. Make healthy choices. Available at: www.cancer.ca/en/prevention-and-screening/reduce-cancer-risk/make-healthy-choices. Accessed June 1, 2018.

Chasan-Taber L, Willett WC, Seddon JM, et al. A prospective study of carotenoid and vitamin A intakes and risk of cataract extraction in US women. *Am J Clin Nutr*, 1999 Oct; 70 (4): 509–16.

Chiu CJ, Milton RC, Gensler G, Taylor A. Dietary carbohydrate intake and glycemic index in relation to cortical and nuclear lens opacities in the Age-Related Eye Disease Study. *Am J Clin Nutr*, 2006 May; 8 (5): 1177–84.

Chiu CJ, Milton RC, Klein R, et al. Dietary carbohydrate and the progression of age-related macular degeneration: A prospective study from the Age-Related Eye Disease Study. *Am J Clin Nutr*, 2007 Oct; 86 (4): 1210–18.

Chuang J, Shih KC, Chan TC, et al. Preoperative optimization of ocular surface disease before cataract surgery. *J Cataract Refract Surg*, 2017 Dec; 43 (12): 1596–1607.

Congdon N, O'Colmain B, Klaver CC, et al; Eye Diseases Prevalence Research Group. Causes and prevalence of visual impairment among adults in the United States. *Arch Ophthalmol*, 2004 Apr; 122 (4): 477–85.

Health Canada. Body mass index (BMI) nomogram. Available at: www.canada.ca/en/health-canada/services/food-nutrition/healthy-eating/healthy-weights/canadian-guidelines-body-weight-classification-adults/body-mass-index-nomogram.html. Accessed June 1, 2018.

Health Canada. A consumer's guide to the DRIs (Dietary Reference Intakes). Available at: www.canada.ca/en/health-canada/services/food-nutrition/healthy-eating/dietary-reference-intakes/consumer-guide-dris-dietary-reference-intakes.html. Accessed June 1, 2018.

Health Canada. Eating well with Canada's food guide. Available at: www.canada.ca/content/dam/hc-sc/migration/hc-sc/fn-an/alt_formats/hpfb-dgpsa/pdf/food-guide-aliment/print_eatwell_bienmang-eng.pdf. Accessed June 1, 2018.

Health Canada. Health effects of ultraviolet radiation. Available at: www.canada.ca/en/health-canada/services/sun-safety/health-effects-ultraviolet-radiation.html. Accessed June 1, 2018.

Health Canada. Mercury in fish. Available at: www.canada.ca/en/health-canada/services/food-nutrition/food-safety/chemical-contaminants/environmental-contaminants/mercury/mercury-fish.html. Accessed June 1, 2018.

Health Canada. Obesity. *It's Your Health*, October 2006. Available at: www.canada.ca/content/dam/hc-sc/migration/hc-sc/hl-vs/alt_formats/pacrb-dgapcr/pdf/iyh-vsv/life-vie/obes-eng.pdf. Accessed June 1, 2018.

Health Canada. Quit smoking. Available at: www.canada.ca/en/health-canada/services/smoking-tobacco/quit-smoking.html. Accessed June 1, 2018.

Klein R, Knudtson MD, Cruickshanks KJ, Klein BE. Further observations on the association between smoking and the long-term incidence and progression of age-related macular degeneration: The Beaver Dam Eye Study. *Arch Ophthalmol*, 2008 Jan; 126 (1): 115–21.

Maxxam Analytics (Mississauga, ON) for the Guelph Food Technology Centre. Commissioned study on the nutrient properties of orange peppers. August 2010.

McDermott JH. Antioxidant nutrients: Current dietary recommendations and research update. *J Am Pharm Assoc* (Wash), 2000 Nov–Dec; 40 (6): 785–99.

Miljanović B, Trivedi KA, Dana MR, et al. Relation between dietary n-3 and n-6 fatty acids and clinically diagnosed dry eye syndrome in women. *Am J Clin Nutr*, 2005 Oct; 82 (4): 887–93.

Moeller SM, Parekh N, Tinker L, et al; CAREDS Research Study Group. Association between intermediate age-related macular degeneration and lutein and zeaxanthin in the Carotenoids in Age-Related Eye Disease Study (CAREDS): Ancillary study of the Women's Health Initiative. *Arch Ophthalmol*, 2006 Aug; 124 (8): 1151–62.

Moeller S, Voland R, Tinker L, et al; CAREDS Study Group; Women's Health Initiative. Associations between age-related nuclear cataract and lutein and zeaxanthin in the diet and serum in the Carotenoids in Age-Related Eye Disease Study, an ancillary study of the Women's Health Initiative. *Arch Ophthalmol*, 2008 Mar; 126 (3): 354–64.

National Institutes of Health, Office of Dietary Supplements. Vitamin D: Fact sheet for health professionals. Available at: https://ods.od.nih.gov/factsheets/VitaminD-HealthProfessional. Accessed June 1, 2018.

National Institutes of Health, Office of Dietary Supplements. Zinc: Fact sheet for health professionals. Available at: https://ods.od.nih.gov/factsheets/Zinc-HealthProfessional. Accessed June 1, 2018.

Oh R. Practical applications of fish oil (omega-3 fatty acids) in primary care. *J Am Board Fam Pract*, 2005 Jan–Feb; 18 (1): 28–36.

Roodenburg AJ, Leenen R, van het Hof KH, et al. Amount of fat in the diet affects bioavailability of lutein esters but not of alpha-carotene, beta-carotene, and vitamin E in humans. *Am J Clin Nutr*, 2000 May; 71 (5): 1187–93.

SanGiovanni JP, Chew EY, Clemons TE, et al; Age-Related Eye Disease Study Research Group. The relationship of dietary lipid intake and age-related macular degeneration in a case-control study: AREDS Report No. 20. *Arch Ophthalmol*, 2007 May; 125 (5): 671–79.

Seddon J. Obesity linked to increased risk of AMD progression. *Ocul-Surg-News*, 2003; 20: Abstract.

Seddon JM. Multivitamin-multimineral supplements and eye disease: Age-related macular degeneration and cataract. *Am J Clin Nutr*, 2007 Jan; 85 (1): 304S–7S.

Seddon JM, Ajani UA, Sperduto RD, et al. Dietary carotenoids, vitamins A, C, and E, and advanced age-related macular degeneration. Eye Disease Case-Control Study Group. *JAMA*, 1994 Nov 9; 272 (18): 1413–20.

Seddon JM, Cote J, Davis N, Rosner B. Progression of age-related macular degeneration: Association with body mass index, waist circumference, and waist-hip ratio. *Arch Ophthalmol*, 2003 Jun; 121 (6): 785–92.

Seddon JM, Cote J, Rosner B. Progression of age-related macular degeneration association with dietary fat, transunsaturated fat, nuts, and fish intake. *Arch Ophthalmol*, 2003 Dec; 121 (12): 1728–37.

Tan AG, Mitchell P, Flood VM, et al. Antioxidant nutrient intake and the long-term incidence of age-related cataract: The Blue Mountains Eye Study. *Am J Clin Nutr*, 2008 Jun; 87 (6): 1899–905.

Tan JS, Wang JJ, Liew G, et al. Age-related macular degeneration and mortality from cardiovascular disease or stroke. *Br J Ophthalmol*, 2008 Apr; 92 (4): 509–12.

Townend BS, Townend ME, Flood V, et al. Dietary macronutrient intake and five-year incident cataract: The Blue Mountains Eye Study. *Am J Ophthalmol*, 2007 Jun; 143 (6): 932–39.

United States Department of Agriculture, Agricultural Research Service. USDA food composition databases. Available at: https://ndb.nal.usda.gov/ndb/search/list. Accessed June 1, 2018.

Chapter 3: Common Eye Conditions and Diseases
Age-Related Macular Degeneration

Age-Related Eye Disease Study Research Group (AREDS). A randomized, placebo-controlled, clinical trial of high-dose supplementation with vitamins C and E, beta carotene, and zinc for age-related macular degeneration and vision loss: AREDS report No.8. *Arch Ophthalmol*, 2001 Oct; 119 (10): 1417–36.

Age-Related Eye Disease Study Research Group (AREDS). The relationship of dietary carotenoid and vitamin A, E, and C intake with age-related macular degeneration in a case-control study: AREDS report No. 22. *Arch Ophthalmol*, 2007 Sep; 125 (9): 1225–32.

Age-Related Eye Disease Study Research Group (AREDS). The relationship of dietary omega-3 long-chain polyunsaturated fatty acid intake with incident age-related macular degeneration: AREDS report No. 23. *Arch Ophthalmol*, 2008 Sep; 126 (9): 1274–79.

Age-Related Eye Disease Study 2 (AREDS2) Research Group. Secondary analyses of the effects of lutein/zeaxanthin on age-related macular degeneration progression: AREDS2 report No. 3. *JAMA Ophthalmol*, 2014 Feb; 132 (2), 142–49.

Age-Related Eye Disease Study 2 (AREDS2). The lutein/zeaxanthin and omega-3 supplementation trial. Available at: www.areds2.org. Accessed June 1, 2018.

Augood C, Chakravarthy U, Young I, et al. Oily fish consumption, dietary docosahexaenoic acid and eicosapentaenoic acid intakes, and associations with neovascular age-related macular degeneration. *Am J Clin Nutr*, 2008 Aug; 88 (2): 398–406.

Awh CC, Zanke B, Kustra R. Progression from no AMD to intermediate AMD as influenced by antioxidant treatment and genetic risk: An analysis of data from the Age-Related Eye Disease Study Cataract Trial. *J Vitreoretin Dis*, 2017 Jan; 1 (1): 45–51.

Awh CC, Hawken S, Zanke BW. Treatment response to antioxidants and zinc based on CFH and ARMS2 genetic risk allele number in the Age-Related Eye Disease Study. *Ophthalmology*, 2015 Jan; 122 (1), 162–69.

Braakhuis A, Raman R, Vaghefi E. The association between dietary intake of antioxidants and ocular disease. *Diseases*, 2017 Jan 30; 5 (1): 3.

Brown DM, Regillo CD. Anti-VEGF agents in the treatment of neovascular age-related macular degeneration: Applying clinical trial results to the treatment of everyday patients. *Am J Ophthalmol*, 2007 Oct; 144 (4): 627–37.

Chew EY. Nutrition, genes, and age-related macular degeneration: What have we learned from the trials? *Ophthalmologica*, 2017; 238 (1–2): 1–5.

Kaushik S, Wang JJ, Flood V, et al. Dietary glycemic index and the risk of age-related macular degeneration. *Am J Clin Nutr*, 2008 Oct; 88 (4): 1104–10.

Korobelnik JF, Rougier MB, Delyfer MN, et al. Effect of dietary supplementation with lutein, zeaxanthin, and ω-3 on macular pigment: A randomized clinical trial. *JAMA Ophthalmol*, 2017 Nov 1; 135 (11): 1259–66.

Lawrenson JG, Evans JR. Omega 3 fatty acids for preventing or slowing the progression of age-related macular degeneration. *Cochrane Database Syst Rev*, 2015 Apr 9; (4): CD010015.

Merle BMJ, Silver RE, Rosner B, Seddon JM. Associations between vitamin D intake and progression to incident advanced age-related macular degeneration. *Invest Ophthalmol Vis Sci*, 2017 Sep 1; 58 (11): 4569–78.

National Eye Institute. Age-related macular degeneration (AMD) tables. Available at: https://nei.nih.gov/eyedata/amd/tables. Accessed June 1, 2018.

Parke DW II. Genetic testing for AMD? An issue settled … for now. *EyeNet Magazine*, July 2017: 14.

Richer S, Ulanski L II, Popenko NA, et al. Age-related macular degeneration beyond the Age-Related Eye Disease Study II. *Adv Ophthalmol Optom*, 2016 Aug; 1 (1): 335–69.

Schwartz SG, Hampton BM, Kovach JL, Brantley MA Jr. Genetics and age-related macular degeneration: A practical review for the clinician. *Clin Ophthalmol*, 2016 Jul 4; 10: 1229–35.

Seddon JM. Macular degeneration epidemiology: Nature-nurture, lifestyle factors, genetic risk, and gene-environment interactions — The Weisenfeld Award Lecture. *Invest Ophthalmol Vis Sci*, 2017 Dec 1; 58 (14): 6513–28.

Somani S, Hoskin-Mott A, Mishra A, et al. Managing patients at risk for age-related macular degeneration: A Canadian strategy. *Can J Optom*, 2009 Mar; 71 (2): 14–20.

Vavvas DG, Small KW, Awh CC, et al. *CFH* and *ARMS2* genetic risk determines progression to neovascular age-related macular degeneration after antioxidant and zinc supplementation. *Proc Natl Acad Sci U S A*, 2018 Jan 23; 115 (4): E696–E704.

Cataracts

Jacques PF, Chylack LT Jr, Hankinson SE, et al. Long-term nutrient intake and early age-related nuclear lens opacities. *Arch Ophthalmol*, 2001 Jul; 119 (7): 1009–19.

Dry Eye Syndrome and Eyelid Disorders

Bron AJ, Tomlinson A, Foulks GN, et al. Rethinking dry eye disease: A perspective on clinical implications. *Ocul Surf*, 2014 Apr; 12 (2 Suppl): S1–31.

Calder PC. N-3 polyunsaturated fatty acids, inflammation, and inflammatory diseases. *Am J Clin Nutr*, 2006 Jun; 83 (6 Suppl): 1505S–19S.

Canadian Association of Optometrists. Screening, diagnosis and management of dry eye disease: Practical guidelines for Canadian optometrists. *National Dry Eye Disease Guidelines for Canadian Optometrists. Can J Optom*, Special Supplement; 76 (Suppl 1).

Craig JP, Nichols KK, Akpek EK, et al. TFOS DEWS II definition and classification report. *Ocul Surf*, 2017 Jul; 15 (3): 276–83.

Liu XF, Hao JL, Xie T, et al. Curcumin, a potential therapeutic candidate for anterior segment eye diseases: A review. *Front Pharmacol*, 2017 Feb 14; 8: 66.

Willcox MDP, Argüeso P, Georgiev GA, et al. TFOS DEWS II tear film report. *Ocul Surf*, 2017 Jul; 15 (3): 366–403.

Wolffsohn JS, Arita R, Chalmers R, et al. TFOS DEWS II diagnostic methodology report. *Ocul Surf*, 2017 Jul; 15 (3): 539–74.

Glaucoma

Al Owaifeer AM, Al Taisan AA. The role of diet in glaucoma: A review of the current evidence. *Ophthalmol Ther*, 2018 Jun; 7 (1): 19–31.

Klein BE, Klein R, Sponsel WE, et al. Prevalence of glaucoma: The Beaver Dam Eye Study. *Ophthalmology*, 1992 Oct; 99 (10): 1499–504.

McMonnies CW. Intraocular pressure and glaucoma: Is physical exercise beneficial or a risk? *J Optom*, 2016 Jul–Sep; 9 (3): 139–47.

Prevent Blindness America. Vision problems in the U.S.: Prevalence of adult vision impairment and age-related eye disease in America. Available at: www.visionproblemsus.org. Accessed June 1, 2018.

Raman R, Vaghefi E, Braakhuis AJ. Food components and ocular pathophysiology: A critical appraisal of the role of oxidative mechanisms. *Asia Pac J Clin Nutr*, 2017; 26 (4): 572–85.

Diabetes

American Diabetes Association. Statistics about diabetes. Available at: www.diabetes.org/diabetes-basics/statistics/?loc=db-slabnav. Accessed June 2018.

Appel LJ, Sacks FM, Carey VJ, et al. Effects of protein, monounsaturated fat, and carbohydrate intake on blood pressure and serum lipids: Results of the OmniHeart randomized trial. *JAMA*, 2005 Nov 16; 294 (19): 2455–64.

Barlow SE; Expert Committee. Expert committee recommendations regarding the prevention, assessment, and treatment of child and adolescent overweight and obesity: Summary report. *Pediatrics*, 2007 Dec; 120 Suppl 4: S164–92.

Bazzano LA, Li TY, Joshipura KJ, Hu FB. Intake of fruit, vegetables and fruit juices and risk of diabetes in women. *Diabetes Care*, 2008 Jul; 31 (7): 1311–17.

Capogna L, Pelletier B. Nutrition and diabetes: Our role in patient care. *Review of Optometry*, 2014 Mar 15. Available at www.reviewofoptometry.com/article/nutrition-and-diabetes-our-role-in-patient-care.

Centers for Disease Control and Prevention. National diabetes fact sheet: National estimates and general information on diabetes and prediabetes in the United States, 2011. Atlanta, GA: U.S. Department of Health and Human Services, Centers for Disease Control and Prevention, 2011. Available at: www.cdc.gov/diabetes/pubs/pdf/ndfs_2011.pdf. Accessed June 1, 2018.

Diabetes Prevention Program Research Group, Knowler WC, Fowler SE, et al. 10-year follow-up of diabetes incidence and weight loss in the Diabetes Prevention Program Outcomes Study. *Lancet*, 2009 Nov 14; 374 (9702): 1677–86.

DiLillo V, Siegfried NJ, West DS. Incorporating motivational interviewing into behavioral obesity treatment. *Cogn Behav Pract*, 2003; 10 (2): 120–30.

Fung TT, Hu FB, Pereira MA, et al. Whole-grain intake and the risk of type 2 diabetes: A prospective study in men. *Am J Clin Nutr*, 2002 Sep; 76 (3): 535–40.

Harvard School of Public Health. Simple steps to preventing diabetes. Available at: www.hsph.harvard.edu/nutritionsource/preventing-diabetes-full-story. Accessed June 1, 2018.

Hu FB, Manson JE, Stampfer MJ, et al. Diet, lifestyle, and the risk of type 2 diabetes mellitus in women. *N Engl J Med*, 2001 Sep 13; 345 (11): 790–97.

International Diabetes Federation. IDF consensus worldwide definition of the metabolic syndrome. Available at: www.idf.org/metabolic-syndrome. Accessed June 1, 2018.

Klein S, Allison DB, Heymsfield SB, et al. Waist circumference and cardiometabolic risk: A consensus statement from Shaping America's Health: Association for Weight Management and Obesity Prevention; NAASO, The Obesity Society; the American Society for Nutrition; and the American Diabetes Association. *Am J Clin Nutr*, 2007 May; 85 (5): 1197–202.

Knowler WC, Barrett-Connor E, Fowler SE, et al. Reduction in the incidence of type 2 diabetes with lifestyle intervention or metformin. *N Engl J Med*, 2002 Feb 7; 346 (6): 393–403.

Liu S, Manson JE, Stampfer MJ, et al. A prospective study of whole-grain intake and risk of type 2 diabetes mellitus in US women. *Am J Public Health*, 2000 Sep; 90 (9): 1409–15.

Mayer-Davis EJ, D'Agostino R Jr, Karter AJ, et al. Intensity and amount of physical activity in relation to insulin sensitivity: The Insulin Resistance Atherosclerosis Study. *JAMA*, 1998 Mar 4; 279 (9): 669–74.

Ogden CL, Carroll MD, Kit BK, Flegal KM. Prevalence of obesity and trends in body mass index among US children and adolescents, 1999–2010. *JAMA*, 2012 Feb 1; 307 (5): 483–90.

Rana JS, Li TY, Manson JE, Hu FB. Adiposity compared with physical inactivity and risk of type 2 diabetes in women. *Diabetes Care*, 2007 Jan; 30 (1): 53–58.

Rosenbloom AL, Silverstein JH, Amemiya S, et al. Type 2 diabetes in children and adolescents. *Pediatr Diabetes*, 2009 Sep; 10 Suppl 12: 17–32.

Schulze MB, Manson JE, Ludwig DS, et al. Sugar-sweetened beverages, weight gain, and incidence of type 2 diabetes in young and middle-aged women. *JAMA*, 2004 Aug 25; 292 (8): 927–34.

SEARCH for Diabetes in Youth Study Group, Liese AD, D'Agostino RB Jr, et al. The burden of diabetes mellitus among US youth: Prevalence estimates from the SEARCH for Diabetes in Youth Study. *Pediatrics*, 2006 Oct; 118 (4): 1510–18.

Wadden TA, Didie E. What's in a name? Patients' preferred terms for describing obesity. *Obes Res*, 2003 Sep; 11 (9): 1140–46.

Yale University: The Rudd Center for Food Policy and Obesity. How to talk about 'weight' with your overweight and obese patients. Available at: www.yaleruddcenter.org/resources/bias_toolkit/toolkit/Module-2/2-01-HowToTalk.pdf. Accessed June 1, 2018.

Chapter 4: Eye Nutrients

Barnett SM, Khan NA, Walk AM, et al. Macular pigment optical density is positively associated with academic performance among preadolescent children. *Nutr Neurosci*, 2018 Nov; 21 (9): 632–40.

Bernstein PS, Li B, Vachali PP, et al. Lutein, zeaxanthin, and meso-zeaxanthin: The basic and clinical science underlying carotenoid-based nutritional interventions against ocular disease. *Prog Retin Eye Res*, 2016 Jan; 50: 34–66.

Carpentier S, Knaus M, Suh M. Associations between lutein, zeaxanthin, and age-related macular degeneration: An overview. *Crit Rev Food Sci Nutr*, 2009 Apr; 49 (4): 313–26.

Cho E, Hung S, Willett WC, et al. Prospective study of dietary fat and the risk of age-related macular degeneration. *Am J Clin Nutr*, 2001 Feb; 73 (2): 209–18.

Chua B, Flood V, Rochtchina E, et al. Dietary fatty acids and the 5-year incidence of age-related maculopathy. *Arch Ophthalmol*, 2006 Jul; 124 (7): 981–86.

Dawe RS. Further evidence for carotenoid antioxidants in photoprotection. *Br J Dermatol*, 2017 May; 176 (5): 1120–21.

Health Canada. Prenatal nutrition guidelines for health professionals: Fish and omega-3 fatty acids. Available at: www.canada.ca/en/health-canada/servicespublications/food-nutrition/prenatal-nutrition-guidelines-health-professionals-fish-omega-3-fatty-acids-2009.html. Accessed June 1, 2018.

Jenkins DJ, Kendall CW, Augustin LS, et al. Glycemic index: Overview of implications in health and disease. *Am J Clin Nutr*, 2002 Jul; 76 (1): 266S–73S.

Jia YP, Sun L, Yu HS, et al. The pharmacological effects of lutein and zeaxanthin on visual disorders and cognition diseases. *Molecules*, 2017 Apr 20; 22 (4). pii: E610.

Johnson EJ, McDonald K, Caldarella SM, et al. Cognitive findings of an exploratory trial of docosahexaenoic acid and lutein supplementation in older women. *Nutr Neurosci*, 2008 Apr; 11 (2): 75–83.

Johnson EJ, Schaefer EJ. Potential role of dietary n-3 fatty acids in the prevention of dementia and macular degeneration. *Am J Clin Nutr*, 2006 Jun; 83 (6 suppl): 1494S–98S.

Ma L, Liu R, Du JH, et al. Lutein, zeaxanthin and meso-zeaxanthin supplementation associated with macular pigment optical density. *Nutrients*, 2016 Jul; 8 (7). pii: E426.

Miller ER 3rd, Pastor-Barriuso R, Dalal D, et al. Meta-analysis: High-dosage vitamin E supplementation may increase all-cause mortality. *Ann Intern Med*, 2005 Jan 4; 142 (1): 37–46.

Morganti P, Bruno C, Guarneri F, et al. Role of topical and nutritional supplement to modify the oxidative stress. *Int J Cosmet Sci*, 2002 Dec; 24 (6): 331–39.

Parekh N, Chappell RJ, Millen AE, et al. Association between vitamin D and age-related macular degeneration in the Third National Health and Nutrition Examination Survey, 1988 through 1994. *Arch Ophthalmol*, 2007 May; 125 (5): 661–69.

Richer S, Stiles W, Statkute L, et al. Double-masked, placebo-controlled, randomized trial of lutein and antioxidant supplementation in the intervention of atrophic age-related macular degeneration: The Veterans LAST Study (Lutein Antioxidant Supplementation Trial). *Optometry*, 2004 Apr; 75 (4): 216–30.

Sato R, Helzlsouer KJ, Alberg AJ, et al. Prospective study of carotenoids, tocopherols, and retinoid concentrations and the risk of breast cancer. *Cancer Epidemiol Biomarkers Prev*, 2002 May; 11 (5): 451–57.

Tan J, Wang JJ, Flood V, et al. Carbohydrate nutrition, glycemic index, and the 10-year incidence of cataract. *Am J Clin Nutr*, 2007 Nov; 86 (5): 1502–8.

Tan JS, Wang JJ, Flood V, et al. Dietary antioxidants and long-term incidence of age-related macular degeneration: The Blue Mountains Eye Study. *Ophthalmology*, 2008 Feb; 115 (2): 334–41.

van der Leun JC. UV radiation from sunlight: Summary, conclusions and recommendations. *J Photochem Photobiol B*, 1996 Sep; 35 (3): 237–44.

Van Leeuwen R, Boekhoorn S, Vingerling J, et al. Dietary intake of antioxidants and risk of age-related macular degeneration. *JAMA*, 2005 Dec 28; 294 (24): 3101–7.

Vishwanathan R, Schalch W, Johnson EJ. Macular pigment carotenoids in the retina and occipital cortex are related in humans. *Nutr Neurosci*, 2016; 19 (3): 95–101.

Voutilainen S, Nurmi T, Mursu J, Rissanen TH. Carotenoids and cardiovascular health. *Am J Clin Nutr*, 2006 Jun; 83 (6): 1265–71.

Chapter 5: Eyefoods

Cackett P, Cheung N, Wong TY. Age-related macular degeneration and mortality from cardiovascular disease or stroke. *Br J Ophthalmol*, 2008 Nov; 92 (11): 1564.

Chitchumroonchokchai C, Schwartz SJ, Failla ML. Assessment of lutein bioavailability from meals and a supplement using simulated digestion and caco-2 human intestinal cells. *J Nutr*, 2004 Sep; 134 (9): 2280–86.

Chung HY, Rasmussen HM, Johnson EJ. Lutein bioavailability is higher from lutein-enriched eggs than from supplements and spinach in men. *J Nutr*, 2004 Aug; 134 (8): 1887–93.

Hu FB, Stampfer MJ, Rimm EB, et al. A prospective study of egg consumption and risk of cardiovascular disease in men and women. *JAMA*, 1999 Apr 21; 281 (15): 1387–94.

National Institutes of Health, Office of Dietary Supplements. Vitamin K Fact Sheet for Consumers. Available at: https://ods.od.nih.gov/pdf/factsheets/VitaminK-Consumer.pdf#search=%22coumadin%22.

Qureshi AI, Suri FK, Ahmed S, et al. Regular egg consumption does not increase the risk of stroke and cardiovascular diseases. *Med Sci Monit*, 2007 Jan; 13 (1): CR1–8.

Chapter 6: Lifestyle and General Health

Drobek-Slowik M, Karczewicz D, Safranow K. The potential role of oxidative stress in the pathogenesis of the age-related macular degeneration (AMD). [Article in Polish.] *Postepy Hig Med Dosw* (Online), 2007; 61: 28–37.

Fletcher AE, Bentham GC, Agnew M, et al. Sunlight exposure, antioxidants, and age-related macular degeneration. *Arch Ophthalmol*, 2008 Oct; 126 (10): 1396–403.

Health Canada. Tanning beds and equipment. Available at: www.canada.ca/en/health-canada/services/sun-safety/tanning-beds-lamps.html. Accessed June 1, 2018.

Tosini G, Ferguson I, Tsubota K. Effects of blue light on the circadian system and eye physiology. *Mol Vis*, 2016 Jan 24; 22: 61–72.

Wong TY, Klein R, Sun C, et al; Atherosclerosis Risk in Communities Study. Age-related macular degeneration and risk for stroke. *Ann Intern Med*, 2006 Jul 18; 145 (2): 98–106.

Chapter 7: Following the Eyefoods Plan

China-Cornell-Oxford Project, Cornell University. Geographic study of mortality, biochemistry, diet and lifestyle in rural China. Archived September 11, 2010, at the Wayback Machine, Clinical Trial Service Unit & Epidemiological Studies Unit, University of Oxford. Accessed February 3, 2011.

Lindeberg S, Cordain L, Boyd Eaton S. Biological and clinical potential of a palaeolithic diet. *J Nutr Environ Med*, 2003 Sep; 13 (3): 149–60.

Index

A

ALA (alpha-linolenic acid), 81–82
allergies, 19, 20, 43, 55
almonds. *See also* nuts
    Chicken and Almond Lettuce
      Wraps, 209
    Crusted Salmon Fillets, 201
    Eyefoods Dinner Salad, 166
AMD (age-related macular
    degeneration), 29–38
    diagnosis, 31–32
    diet and, 36, 37
    lifestyle and, 35
    overweight and, 31, 110
    risk factors, 31, 34
    symptoms, 30
    treatments, 34
    visual aids for, 36–37
amino acids, 71
Amsler grid, 31–32
angiography, 33
antioxidants, 75
apricots
    Chicken and Lentil Salad with
      Mint, 170
    Eyefoods Trail Mix, 222
    Kale Salad with Chickpeas, 164
    Mixed Green Salad with Berries
      and Apricots, 154
    Wheat Berry and Apricot Salad,
      162
aqueous humor, 10
arugula, 85
    Awesome Arugula Chopped
      Salad, 155
astigmatism, 12
avocados
    Avocado Salad with Radishes,
      159
    Eggs Benny with Roasted Pepper
      Coulis, 129
    Green Smoothie Bowl, 132
    Lentil and Avocado Salad, 168

B

Balsamic Vinaigrette, 171
bananas
    Banana Matcha Green Smoothie,
      144
    Berry Banana Green Smoothie,
      140
    Chocolate Goji Berry Green
      Smoothie, 144
    Chocolate Smoothie Bowl, 133
    Green Smoothie Bowl, 132
    Melon Mint Green Smoothie, 141
    Pumpkin Pie Smoothie, 148
    Vanilla Pear Green Smoothie, 141

barley, 100
    Beef and Broccoli with Barley,
      219
    Stuffed Orange Peppers, 217
    Turkey, Pea and Carrot Barley
      Bowls, 213
Basic Salad Dressing, 171
beans, 102–3. *See also* beans, green;
    chickpeas; edamame
    Black Bean and Mango Salad, 165
    Carrot and Romano Bean Salad,
      167
    Chicken and Black Bean Rice
      Bowls with Wasabi Lime
      Sauce, 210
    Deli-Style Kale Salad, 167
    Eyefoods Dinner Salad, 166
    Kale and White Bean Soup, 190
    Rapini with White Beans and
      Red Pepper, 183
    Turkey and Orange Pepper Chili
      with Lime, 194
    Turkey Fajitas, 212
    White Bean Dip, 227
beans, green
    Green Salad with Herbs, 153
    Niçoise Salad, 156
beef
    Beef and Broccoli with Barley,
      219
    Mango and Beef Stir-Fry, 220
    Mom's Eye-Friendly Meatloaf,
      218
    Stuffed Orange Peppers, 217
berries. *See also* goji berries
    Berry Banana Green Smoothie,
      140
    Chocolate Smoothie Bowl, 133
    Coconut Berry Smoothie, 146
    Kiwi, Mango and Blackberry
      Fruit Bowl, 134
    Mixed Green Salad with Berries
      and Apricots, 154
    Strawberry, Watermelon and
      Mint Smoothie, 146
beta-carotene, 75–76
Beta-Carotene Blast, 149
beverages, 66, 95–96, 137
blepharitis, 50–51
blink rate, 108
blue light exposure, 105–9
BMI (body mass index), 110.
    See also overweight
bran
    Crusted Salmon Fillets, 201
    Pumpkin Savory Loaf, 131
breakfasts, 126–34
breast milk, 16

broccoli, 93
    Beef and Broccoli with Barley,
      219
    Broccoli, Edamame and Nut Rice
      Bowls, 197
    Broccoli and Orange Pepper
      Salad, 160
    Broccoli and Spinach Soup, 180
    Chicken and Black Bean Rice
      Bowls with Wasabi Lime
      Sauce, 210
    Green Salad with Herbs, 153
    Shrimp Stir-Fry, 206
    Turkey Stir-Fry with Peanut
      Sauce, 211
broccoli, Chinese (gai lan), 85
buckwheat, 101
bulgur, 101

C

cabbage, 85
    Sautéed Savoy Cabbage, 184
cannabis, 59–60
cantaloupe. *See* melons
carbohydrates, 68–71
cardiovascular disease, 25, 60, 99,
    111
carotenoids, 75
carrots, 91
    Beta-Carotene Blast, 149
    Broccoli and Orange Pepper
      Salad, 160
    Broccoli and Spinach Soup, 180
    Carrot and Romano Bean Salad,
      167
    Carrot Fries, 185
    Carrot Mango Smoothie, 148
    Deli-Style Kale Salad, 167
    Lentil Soup, 191
    Sweet Potato and Lentil Stew, 193
    Sweet Potato and Orange Pepper
      Soup, 181
    Turkey, Pea and Carrot Barley
      Bowls, 213
cataracts, 38–41
Cauliflower, Roasted Butternut
    Squash and, 186
celery
    Broccoli and Spinach Soup, 180
    Lentil Soup, 191
    Sweet Potato and Orange Pepper
      Soup, 181
chalazia, 50
cheese
    Crustless Quiche, 199
    Greek-Style Corn Salad, 163
    Mom's Eye-Friendly Meatloaf, 218
    Sweet Potato and Kale Bake, 198

cheese (*continued*)
Turkey Meatballs in Tomato Sauce, 216
Whole Wheat Penne with Spinach, 195
chicken. *See also* turkey
Chicken and Almond Lettuce Wraps, 209
Chicken and Black Bean Rice Bowls with Wasabi Lime Sauce, 210
Chicken and Lentil Salad with Mint, 170
Chicken Cacciatore, 208
chickpeas. *See also* beans
Greek-Style Corn Salad, 163
Hummus, 226
Kale Salad with Chickpeas, 164
Pumpkin Hummus, 227
children, 16–18, 106
chocolate. *See* cocoa powder
cholesterol, 73, 94
choroid, 10
Citrus Dressing, 172
Citrus Mint Salsa, 187
Citrus Zinger, 150
cocoa powder
Chocolate Goji Berry Green Smoothie, 144
Chocolate Smoothie Bowl, 133
Turkey and Orange Pepper Chili with Lime, 194
coconut milk beverage
Berry Banana Green Smoothie, 140
Carrot Mango Smoothie, 148
Chocolate Goji Berry Green Smoothie, 144
Coconut Berry Smoothie, 146
Mango, Mint and Lime Green Smoothie, 142
coconut water
Goji Berry Smoothie, 147
Green Smoothie Bowl, 132
Strawberry, Watermelon and Mint Smoothie, 146
Tropical Eye Power Green Smoothie, 143
collard greens, 85. *See also* greens
computers. *See* screen time
conjunctiva, 9
contact lenses, 19, 22, 44, 47.
See also refractive errors
corn
Edamame and Pepper Salad with Kalamata Olives, 168
Greek-Style Corn Salad, 163
Turkey Fajitas, 212
cornea, 10, 50
Crab, Orecchiette with Baby Peas and, 204
Creamy Miso Dressing, 173
Creamy Salad Dressing, 172

Create-Your-Own Mason Jar Salad, 152
cucumber
Avocado Salad with Radishes, 159
Goji Berry Smoothie, 147
Strawberry, Watermelon and Mint Smoothie, 146
curcumin, 46

D
dandelion greens, 84. *See also* greens
Deli-Style Kale Salad, 167
demodex (mites), 45, 51
desserts, 228–29
DHA (docosahexaenoic acid), 16, 19, 81–82
diabetes, 61–66
diet and, 65–66
ocular effects, 63–65
diet. *See also* eyefoods
and AMD, 36, 37
and dry eye syndrome, 47, 48–49
and glaucoma, 58–59
sugar in, 66, 69–70
supplements and, 79
Dillicious Spinach Frittata, 128
dips, 226–27
Dr. Barb's Green Smoothie, 139
DRIs (dietary reference intakes), 69
dry eye syndrome, 24, 41–49
diagnosis, 45–46
diet and, 47, 48–49
risk factors, 43–45
treatments, 46–49

E
edamame
Broccoli, Edamame and Nut Rice Bowls, 197
Edamame and Pepper Salad with Kalamata Olives, 168
Turkey and Mango Orange Pepper Boats, 179
eggs, 94, 119
Crustless Quiche, 199
Dillicious Spinach Frittata, 128
Eggs Benny with Roasted Pepper Coulis, 129
Eyefoods Dinner Salad, 166
Niçoise Salad, 156
Orange Pepper, Spinach and Sun-Dried Tomato Frittata, 127
Perfect Poached Eggs, 129
Sabayon with Fresh Fruit, 229
Turkey Meatballs in Tomato Sauce, 216
EPA (eicosapentaenoic acid), 81–82
exercise, 25, 63, 111, 116
eye care, 16–27
for babies, 17

for children, 16–18
for the elderly, 25–27
in middle age, 21–23
for preschoolers, 18
for seniors, 23–25
for teens, 19
for young adults, 20–21
eye drops, 19, 22, 50
diagnostic, 45
for dry eye syndrome, 46, 48
for glaucoma, 55, 56, 58
eye examinations, 9, 14, 28
eyefoods
for diabetes, 66
and lifestyle, 116
meal plans, 122–24
for nutrition, 112–15
for paleo diet, 117–18
pantry staples, 124
for plant-based diet, 118–19
for preschoolers, 18
tips, 120
tracking intake, 121
eyelid disorders, 50–51
eye makeup, 45
eyes
anatomy, 8–11
color of, 16
nutrients for, 14–15, 74, 113
refractive errors of, 12–13, 63

F
Fajitas, Turkey, 212
farro, 101
fat (dietary), 71–73, 104
fennel (bulb)
Citrus Mint Salsa, 187
Poached Salmon, 200
Roasted Butternut Squash and Cauliflower, 186
fiber (dietary), 70–71, 81
fish and seafood, 87–90
Awesome Arugula Chopped Salad, 155
Crusted Salmon Fillets, 201
Eyefoods Dinner Salad, 166
Grilled Scallop and Pineapple Skewers, 205
Mango Tango Salmon, 202
Niçoise Salad, 156
Orecchiette with Baby Peas and Crab, 204
Poached Salmon, 200
Rainbow Trout Packets, 203
Shrimp Stir-Fry, 206
flax seeds, 101. *See also* seeds
floaters, 10
fovea, 11
fruit, 95. *See also* berries; fruit, dried; *specific fruits*
Green Smoothie Bowl, 132
Sabayon with Fresh Fruit, 229
water infused with, 137

fruit, dried. *See also* goji berries
    Deli-Style Kale Salad, 167
    Eyefoods Granola, 223
    Eyefoods Trail Mix, 222
    Kale Salad with Chickpeas, 164

G

gai lan (Chinese broccoli), 85
garlic
    Kale Pesto, 188
    Orange Curry Dressing, 173
gingerroot
    Beef and Broccoli with Barley, 219
    Broccoli, Edamame and Nut Rice
      Bowls, 197
    Mango and Beef Stir-Fry, 220
    Pear, Ginger and Mint Juice, 150
    Shrimp Stir-Fry, 206
    Sweet Potato and Orange Pepper
      Soup, 181
    Turkey, Pea and Carrot Barley
      Bowls, 213
glasses, 21, 109. *See also* sunglasses
glaucoma, 52–60
    cannabis and, 59–60
    diagnosis, 53–55
    diet and, 58–59
    narrow-angle, 56–58
    normal-tension, 56
    primary open-angle, 52–56
    risk factors, 53, 57
    secondary, 58
    symptoms, 57
    treatments, 55–56, 58
glycemic index/load, 70
goji berries (dried)
    Chocolate Goji Berry Green
      Smoothie, 144
    Eyefoods Fruit Salad, 134
    Eyefoods Trail Mix, 222
    Goji Berry Smoothie, 147
    Green Smoothie Bowl, 132
    Mixed Green Salad with Berries
      and Apricots, 154
grains, 65, 99–102. *See also specific*
    grains
    cooking, 178
    gluten-free, 100
grapefruit
    Beta-Carotene Blast, 149
    Citrus Mint Salsa, 187
    Citrus Zinger, 150
    Pear, Ginger and Mint Juice, 150
grapes
    Dr. Barb's Green Smoothie, 139
    Eyefoods Fruit Salad, 134
    Peach Grape Green Smoothie,
      140
Greek-Style Corn Salad, 163
greens (leafy), 83–87. *See also*
    specific greens
    Chocolate Goji Berry Green
      Smoothie, 144

Mix-and-Match Sautéed Greens,
    176
Sautéed Greens with Sweet
    Potato and Pear, 182
Shrimp Stir-Fry, 206

H

herbs (fresh). *See also* mint
    Eyefoods Shepherd's Pie, 214
    Green Salad with Herbs, 153
    Kale and White Bean Soup, 190
    Kale Pesto, 188
    Kale Soup with Turkey and Wild
      Rice, 192
    Mango and Beef Stir-Fry, 220
    Poached Salmon, 200
    Sweet Potato and Kale Bake, 198
    water infused with, 137
high blood pressure, 60
Hummus, 226
hyperopia (farsightedness), 12

I

inflammation (chronic), 51
insulin, 62
IOP (intraocular pressure), 52–53.
    See also glaucoma
iris, 10

J

juices, 95–96, 136–37
    recipes, 149–50

K

kale, 84. *See also* greens; spinach
    Berry Banana Green Smoothie,
      140
    Chocolate Smoothie Bowl, 133
    Crustless Quiche, 199
    Deli-Style Kale Salad, 167
    Dr. Barb's Green Smoothie, 139
    Kale and Sweet Potato Hash, 130
    Kale and White Bean Soup, 190
    Kale Chips, 223
    Kale Pesto, 188
    Kale Salad with Chickpeas, 164
    Kale Soup with Turkey and Wild
      Rice, 192
    Kiwi Mango Green Smoothie, 142
    Mango, Mint and Lime Green
      Smoothie, 142
    Mediterranean-Style Kale Salad,
      158
    Melon Matcha Green Smoothie,
      145
    Melon Mint Green Smoothie, 141
    Nutty Kale Chips, 224
    Orange Kiwi Green Smoothie,
      143
    Orange Pepper and Kale Tossed
      Salad, 157
    Peach Grape Green Smoothie, 140
    Pear, Ginger and Mint Juice, 150

Rainbow Trout Packets, 203
Seedy Kale Chips, 225
Sweet Potato and Kale Bake, 198
Vanilla Pear Green Smoothie, 141
kiwifruit
    Dr. Barb's Green Smoothie, 139
    Eyefoods Fruit Salad, 134
    Kiwi, Mango and Blackberry
      Fruit Bowl, 134
    Kiwi Mango Green Smoothie, 142
    Orange Kiwi Green Smoothie,
      143

L

lemon
    Basic Salad Dressing, 171
    Citrus Dressing, 172
    Citrus Zinger, 150
    Orecchiette with Baby Peas and
      Crab, 204
lens, 10. *See also* cataracts
lentils, 71, 102–3. *See also* beans
    Chicken and Lentil Salad with
      Mint, 170
    Lentil and Avocado Salad, 168
    Lentil and Orange Salad, 169
    Lentil Soup, 191
    Sweet Potato and Lentil Stew, 193
lettuce, 85, 86
    Chicken and Almond Lettuce
      Wraps, 209
    Eyefoods Dinner Salad, 166
    Green Salad with Herbs, 153
    Mixed Green Salad with Berries
      and Apricots, 154
    Niçoise Salad, 156
lifestyle, 105–11, 116
lime
    Banana Matcha Green Smoothie,
      144
    Beta-Carotene Blast, 149
    Chicken and Black Bean Rice
      Bowls with Wasabi Lime
      Sauce, 210
    Citrus Mint Salsa, 187
    Citrus Zinger, 150
    Eyefoods Fruit Salad, 134
    Mango Tango Salmon, 202
    Nutty Kale Chips, 224
    Rainbow Trout Packets, 203
    Strawberry, Watermelon and
      Mint Smoothie, 146
    Turkey and Orange Pepper Chili
      with Lime, 194
lutein, 26, 76–77

M

macronutrients, 68–73. *See also*
    specific nutrients
macula, 11, 65, 77. *See also* AMD
mangos
    Black Bean and Mango Salad, 165
    Carrot Mango Smoothie, 148

mangos (continued)
  Goji Berry Smoothie, 147
  Kiwi, Mango and Blackberry
    Fruit Bowl, 134
  Kiwi Mango Green Smoothie,
    142
  Mango, Mint and Lime Green
    Smoothie, 142
  Mango and Beef Stir-Fry, 220
  Mango Spinach Salad, 158
  Mango Tango Salmon, 202
  Tropical Eye Power Green
    Smoothie, 143
  Turkey and Mango Orange
    Pepper Boats, 179
maple syrup
  Eyefoods Granola, 223
  Not-So-Green Smoothie for
    Beginners, 138
  Pumpkin Mousse, 228
  Sabayon with Fresh Fruit, 229
Mason Jar Salad, Create-Your-Own,
  152
matcha powder
  Banana Matcha Green Smoothie,
    144
  Green Smoothie Bowl, 132
  Melon Matcha Green Smoothie,
    145
mayonnaise
  Creamy Miso Dressing, 173
  Creamy Salad Dressing, 172
meal plans, 65, 122–24
Mediterranean-Style Kale Salad,
  158
Meibomian glands, 10, 41–42, 46,
  47. See also dry eye syndrome
  inflammation of (meibomianitis),
  50–51
melons
  Cantaloupe Drinkable Yogurt,
    149
  Eyefoods Fruit Salad, 134
  Melon Matcha Green Smoothie,
    145
  Melon Mint Green Smoothie, 141
  Strawberry, Watermelon and
    Mint Smoothie, 146
mercury, 89
meso-zeaxanthin, 77
micronutrients, 73–82. See also
  specific nutrients
milk (non-dairy). See also coconut
  milk beverage
  Berry Banana Green Smoothie,
    140
  Broccoli and Spinach Soup, 180
  Chocolate Goji Berry Green
    Smoothie, 144
  Chocolate Smoothie Bowl, 133
  Pumpkin Pie Smoothie, 148
  Vanilla Pear Green Smoothie,
    141

mint. See also herbs
  Chicken and Lentil Salad with
    Mint, 170
  Citrus Mint Salsa, 187
  Mango, Mint and Lime Green
    Smoothie, 142
  Melon Mint Green Smoothie,
    141
  Pear, Ginger and Mint Juice, 150
  Strawberry, Watermelon and
    Mint Smoothie, 146
Miso Dressing, Creamy, 173
Mix-and-Match Sautéed Greens,
  176
Mom's Eye-Friendly Meatloaf, 218
myopia (nearsightedness), 12

N
nerves, 11
Niçoise Salad, 156
noodles. See pasta and noodles
Not-So-Green Smoothie for
  Beginners, 138
nuts, 98–99. See also almonds; nut
  butters
  Broccoli, Edamame and Nut Rice
    Bowls, 197
  Chocolate Smoothie Bowl, 133
  Eyefoods Granola, 223
  Eyefoods Nut Mix, 222
  Eyefoods Trail Mix, 222
  Nutty Kale Chips, 224
  Orange Pepper and Kale Tossed
    Salad, 157
  Turkey Stir-Fry with Peanut
    Sauce, 211
  Wheat Berry and Apricot Salad,
    162
nut butters
  Chicken and Almond Lettuce
    Wraps, 209
  Turkey Stir-Fry with Peanut
    Sauce, 211
nutrients, 15, 68–82
  DRIs (dietary reference intakes),
    69
  for eye health, 14–15, 74, 113
  as supplements, 79
nutritional yeast
  Nutty Kale Chips, 224
  Seedy Kale Chips, 225

O
oats (rolled), 101
  Eyefoods Granola, 223
  Pumpkin Savory Loaf, 131
obesity. See overweight
olive oil, 104
olives
  Chicken Cacciatore, 208
  Edamame and Pepper Salad
    with Kalamata Olives, 168
  Kale Salad with Chickpeas, 164

Niçoise Salad, 156
Orange Pepper and Kale Tossed
  Salad, 157
Pasta with Rapini, 196
omega-3 fatty acids, 19, 47, 81–82,
  119
omega-6 fatty acids, 82
onions
  Deli-Style Kale Salad, 167
  Greek-Style Corn Salad, 163
  Mango and Beef Stir-Fry, 220
  Mediterranean-Style Kale Salad,
    158
  Turkey Fajitas, 212
optic nerve, 11. See also glaucoma
orange
  Chicken and Almond Lettuce
    Wraps, 209
  Citrus Dressing, 172
  Citrus Mint Salsa, 187
  Citrus Zinger, 150
  Creamy Miso Dressing, 173
  Eyefoods Dinner Salad, 166
  Lentil and Orange Salad, 169
  Not-So-Green Smoothie for
    Beginners, 138
  Orange Curry Dressing, 173
  Orange Kiwi Green Smoothie,
    143
  Peach, Pineapple and Pepper
    Smoothie, 147
  Pumpkin Mousse, 228
  Rainbow Trout Packets, 203
  Sweet Potato and Orange Pepper
    Soup, 181
Orecchiette with Baby Peas and
  Crab, 204
osmolarity, 46
overweight, 31, 62, 65, 110
oxidation, 75

P
paleo diet, 117–18
pasta and noodles
  Orecchiette with Baby Peas
    and Crab, 204
  Pasta with Rapini, 196
  Shrimp Stir-Fry, 206
  Whole Wheat Penne with
    Spinach, 195
PCBs, 89
peaches
  Not-So-Green Smoothie for
    Beginners, 138
  Peach, Pineapple and Pepper
    Smoothie, 147
  Peach Grape Green Smoothie,
    140
pears
  Pear, Ginger and Mint Juice, 150
  Sautéed Greens with Sweet
    Potato and Pear, 182
  Vanilla Pear Green Smoothie, 141

peas (green) and pea shoots, 85
  Chicken and Almond Lettuce
    Wraps, 209
  Chicken and Black Bean Rice
    Bowls with Wasabi Lime
    Sauce, 210
  Eggs Benny with Roasted Pepper
    Coulis, 129
  Eyefoods Dinner Salad, 166
  Eyefoods Shepherd's Pie, 214
  Mango Spinach Salad, 158
  Orecchiette with Baby Peas and
    Crab, 204
  Quinoa and Green Pea Salad, 161
  Turkey, Pea and Carrot Barley
    Bowls, 213
  Turkey Stir-Fry with Peanut
    Sauce, 211
peppers, bell. See also peppers,
    orange
  Black Bean and Mango Salad,
    165
  Carrot and Romano Bean Salad,
    167
  Chicken Cacciatore, 208
  Crustless Quiche, 199
  Edamame and Pepper Salad
    with Kalamata Olives, 168
  Greek-Style Corn Salad, 163
  Green Salad with Herbs, 153
  Kale Salad with Chickpeas, 164
  Lentil and Avocado Salad, 168
  Lentil and Orange Salad, 169
  Orecchiette with Baby Peas and
    Crab, 204
  Pickled Peppers, 225
  Rapini with White Beans and
    Red Pepper, 183
  Roasted Pepper Coulis, 187
  Sweet Potato and Lentil Stew, 193
  Turkey Fajitas, 212
  Turkey Stir-Fry with Peanut
    Sauce, 211
peppers, orange (bell), 92
  Broccoli and Orange Pepper
    Salad, 160
  Chicken and Almond Lettuce
    Wraps, 209
  Chicken and Black Bean Rice
    Bowls with Wasabi Lime
    Sauce, 210
  Dillicious Spinach Frittata, 128
  Eyefoods Dinner Salad, 166
  Mango and Beef Stir-Fry, 220
  Mango Tango Salmon, 202
  Mediterranean-Style Kale Salad,
    158
  Mini Pepper Sailboats, 226
  Mixed Green Salad with Berries
    and Apricots, 154
  Orange Pepper, Spinach and
    Sun-Dried Tomato Frittata,
    127

Orange Pepper and Kale Tossed
    Salad, 157
Peach, Pineapple and Pepper
    Smoothie, 147
Quinoa and Green Pea Salad, 161
Shrimp Stir-Fry, 206
Stuffed Orange Peppers, 217
Sweet Potato and Orange Pepper
    Soup, 181
Turkey and Mango Orange
    Pepper Boats, 179
Turkey and Orange Pepper Chili
    with Lime, 194
Turkey Burgers with Roasted
    Orange Peppers, 215
phytonutrients, 73
pineapple
  Green Smoothie Bowl, 132
  Grilled Scallop and Pineapple
    Skewers, 205
  Peach, Pineapple and Pepper
    Smoothie, 147
  Tropical Eye Power Green
    Smoothie, 143
pine nuts
  Kale Pesto, 188
  Mediterranean-Style Kale Salad,
    158
plant-based diets, 118–19
prediabetes, 61
presbyopia, 12–13, 21
protein, 71, 96–97
pumpkin purée
  Chicken Cacciatore, 208
  Kale and White Bean Soup, 190
  Lentil Soup, 191
  Mango Spinach Salad, 158
  Pumpkin Dressing, 174
  Pumpkin Hummus, 227
  Pumpkin Mousse, 228
  Pumpkin Pie Smoothie, 148
  Pumpkin Savory Loaf, 131
  Sweet Potato and Lentil Stew, 193
pupil, 10

Q
Quiche, Crustless, 199
quinoa, 101
  Quinoa and Green Pea Salad, 161

R
radicchio, 85
  Mixed Green Salad with Berries
    and Apricots, 154
Radishes, Avocado Salad with, 159
Rainbow Trout Packets, 203
rapini, 86
  Pasta with Rapini, 196
  Rapini with White Beans and
    Red Pepper, 183
reading glasses, 14, 21
refractive errors, 12–13, 63
retina, 11, 64

rice and wild rice, 100
  Broccoli, Edamame and Nut Rice
    Bowls, 197
  Chicken and Black Bean Rice
    Bowls with Wasabi Lime
    Sauce, 210
  Kale and White Bean Soup, 190
  Kale Soup with Turkey and Wild
    Rice, 192

S
Sabayon with Fresh Fruit, 229
salad dressings, 171–74
salads, 152–70
salmon, 88
  Crusted Salmon Fillets, 201
  Mango Tango Salmon, 202
  Poached Salmon, 200
sardines, 88
  Awesome Arugula Chopped
    Salad, 155
  Niçoise Salad, 156
sclera, 9
screen time, 44–45, 108–9. See also
    blue light exposure
seaweed, 119
seeds, 98–99. See also pine nuts
  Chocolate Smoothie Bowl, 133
  Coconut Berry Smoothie, 146
  Eyefoods Dinner Salad, 166
  Eyefoods Nut Mix, 222
  Green Smoothie Bowl, 132
  Mixed Green Salad with Berries
    and Apricots, 154
  Quinoa and Green Pea Salad, 161
  Seedy Kale Chips, 225
serving sizes, 65, 66, 114
shrimp. See fish and seafood
Sjogren's syndrome, 44
smoking, 31, 51, 60, 110, 116
smoothie bowls, 132–33, 136
smoothies, 136
  fruit and veggie, 146–49
  green, 138–45
snacks, 18, 222–27
soups, 180–81, 190–92
spinach, 84. See also greens; kale
  Awesome Arugula Chopped
    Salad, 155
  Banana Matcha Green Smoothie,
    144
  Broccoli and Spinach Soup, 180
  Chicken and Black Bean Rice
    Bowls with Wasabi Lime
    Sauce, 210
  Dillicious Spinach Frittata, 128
  Eggs Benny with Roasted Pepper
    Coulis, 129
  Eyefoods Dinner Salad, 166
  Eyefoods Shepherd's Pie, 214
  Green Salad with Herbs, 153
  Green Smoothie Bowl, 132
  Lentil Soup, 191

spinach (*continued*)
   Mango Spinach Salad, 158
   Mom's Eye-Friendly Meatloaf, 218
   Niçoise Salad, 156
   Not-So-Green Smoothie for
      Beginners, 138
   Orange Pepper, Spinach and Sun-
      Dried Tomato Frittata, 127
   Stuffed Orange Peppers, 217
   Sweet Potato and Lentil Stew, 193
   Tropical Eye Power Green
      Smoothie, 143
   Whole Wheat Penne with
      Spinach, 195
squash, 91. *See also* pumpkin purée;
   zucchini
   Roasted Butternut Squash and
      Cauliflower, 186
starches, 70
sties, 50
Strawberry, Watermelon and Mint
   Smoothie, 146
sunglasses, 18, 20–21, 106–8
supplements, 79
surgery
   for cataracts, 40
   and dry eye syndrome, 44
   for glaucoma, 56
sweet potatoes, 91
   Chocolate Smoothie Bowl, 133
   Eyefoods Shepherd's Pie, 214
   Kale and Sweet Potato Hash, 130
   Sautéed Greens with Sweet
      Potato and Pear, 182
   Sweet Potato and Kale Bake, 198
   Sweet Potato and Lentil Stew, 193
   Sweet Potato and Orange Pepper
      Soup, 181
Swiss chard, 86. *See also* greens

T

tear film, 9, 42. *See also* dry eye
   syndrome
teenagers, 19
tomatoes and tomato sauce. *See also*
   tomatoes, sun-dried
   Avocado Salad with Radishes, 159
   Chicken Cacciatore, 208
   Kale and Sweet Potato Hash, 130
   Lentil Soup, 191
   Mango Tango Salmon, 202

Stuffed Orange Peppers, 217
Sweet Potato and Kale Bake, 198
Sweet Potato and Lentil Stew, 193
Turkey and Orange Pepper Chili
   with Lime, 194
Turkey Meatballs in Tomato
   Sauce, 216
tomatoes, sun-dried
   Mediterranean-Style Kale Salad,
      158
   Orange Pepper, Spinach and Sun-
      Dried Tomato Frittata, 127
   Quinoa and Green Pea Salad, 161
   Wheat Berry and Apricot Salad,
      162
   White Bean Dip, 227
trans fats, 73
Tropical Eye Power Green
   Smoothie, 143
tuna, 90
turkey. *See also* chicken
   Eyefoods Dinner Salad, 166
   Eyefoods Shepherd's Pie, 214
   Kale Soup with Turkey and Wild
      Rice, 192
   Mom's Eye-Friendly Meatloaf, 218
   Stuffed Orange Peppers, 217
   Turkey, Pea and Carrot Barley
      Bowls, 213
   Turkey and Mango Orange
      Pepper Boats, 179
   Turkey and Orange Pepper Chili
      with Lime, 194
   Turkey Burgers with Roasted
      Orange Peppers, 215
   Turkey Fajitas, 212
   Turkey Meatballs in Tomato
      Sauce, 216
   Turkey Stir-Fry with Peanut
      Sauce, 211

U

ultraviolet (UV) radiation, 105–9

V

Vanilla Pear Green Smoothie, 141
vegetables. *See also* greens; *specific*
   vegetables
   green, 93
   leafy green, 83–87, 109
   orange, 90–91

roasting, 177
   water infused with, 137
vegetarian/vegan diets, 118–19
vision, 12–15
   aids for, 24, 36–37
   loss of, 64
visual field testing, 54
vitamin A. *See* beta-carotene
vitamin C (ascorbic acid), 73, 78
vitamin D, 78–79
vitamin E, 79–80
vitreous humor, 10

W

watercress, 86
wheat berries, 101
   Wheat Berry and Apricot Salad,
      162
wheat germ
   Crusted Salmon Fillets, 201
   Eyefoods Granola, 223
   Nutty Kale Chips, 224
   Seedy Kale Chips, 225
   Turkey Meatballs in Tomato
      Sauce, 216
wine
   Broccoli and Spinach Soup, 180
   Chicken Cacciatore, 208
   Kale and White Bean Soup, 190
   Lentil Soup, 191
   Poached Salmon, 200
   Sabayon with Fresh Fruit, 229
   Sweet Potato and Lentil Stew, 193
   Sweet Potato and Orange Pepper
      Soup, 181

Y

yeast. *See* nutritional yeast
yogurt
   Cantaloupe Drinkable Yogurt,
      149
   Creamy Miso Dressing, 173
   Creamy Salad Dressing, 172
   Orange Curry Dressing, 173
   Pumpkin Mousse, 228

Z

zeaxanthin, 26, 76–77
zinc, 80
zucchini, 93
   Mini Pepper Sailboats, 226

Library and Archives Canada Cataloguing in Publication

Title: Eyefoods : the complete eye health & nutrition guide / Laurie Capogna, OD.

Other titles: Eyefoods (2019) | Complete eye health & nutrition guide | Complete eye health and nutrition guide

Names: Capogna, Laurie, 1973- author.

Description: Includes index.

Identifiers: Canadiana 20190055340 | ISBN 9780778806233 (softcover)

Subjects: LCSH: Eye—Diseases—Nutritional aspects—Popular works. | LCSH: Eye—Diseases—Diet therapy—Popular works. |
     LCSH: Eye—Diseases—Prevention—Popular works. | LCSH: Eye—Care and hygiene—Popular works.

Classification: LCC RE51 .C37 2019 | DDC 617.7/0654—dc23